Coping
With
Rheumatoid
Arthritis

Coping With Rheumatoid Arthritis

Robert H. Phillips, Ph.D.

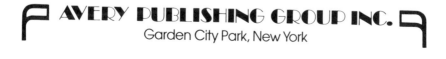

AVERY PUBLISHING GROUP INC.
Garden City Park, New York

The medical information and procedures contained in this book are not intended as a substitute for consulting your physician. All matters regarding your physical health should be supervised by a medical professional.

Cover art by Tim Peterson
Cover design by Martin Hochberg and Rudy Shur
In-house editor Jacqueline Balla
Typesetting by Multifacit Graphics, Aberdeen, NJ

Library of Congress Cataloging-in-Publication Data

Phillips, Robert H., 1948-
    Coping with rheumatoid arthritis.

    Bibliography: p.
    Includes index.
    1. Rheumatoid arthritis–Popular works.
2. Rheumatoid arthritis–Psychological aspects.
3. Rheumatoid arthritis–Social aspects.   I. Title.
RC933.P455   1988   616.7'22   88-3450
ISBN 0-89529-371-4 (pbk.)

Printed in the United States of America

10 9 8 7 6 5 4

Contents

Dedication

In order to cope most effectively, one benefits from the love and support of "significant others." I am, therefore, most grateful to the following special people, to whom this book is dedicated: to my wife, Sharon; my three sons, Michael, Larry, and Steven; my parents; my sister; my grandparents; all my other relatives and in-laws; and my friends.

Acknowledgements

I'd like to express appreciative words of thanks to some wonderful people who provided valuable assistance in the preparation of this book. Thanks to Robert Marcus, M.D., for his critical review, helpful suggestions and information, and enthusiastic participation in this project. Thanks to Jo Wagner for much information, support, and belief in the need for this book. Thanks to William Given, M.D., for his insightful review of the manuscript. Thanks to Sharon Balaban for the long hours spent painstakingly transcribing, revising, and typing the final manuscript. Thanks to Rudy Shur and Jackie Balla for their untiring support and professionalism. Finally, much thanks to Robert Lahita, M.D., Ph.D., for his professional evaluation and overall review—his expertise, judgment, and friendship are highly valued.

Foreword

There are only a few diseases in the world which affect great numbers of people. One particularly common disease in this group is rheumatoid arthritis. This illness has afflicted man since antiquity, for which no cause is known, and for which there is no cure. Despite this, rheumatoid arthritis is not terminal, but rather a long-term illness which cripples many, causes intense worry for most others, and changes the way those who get it perceive their lives, their work, and their relationships with others. Certainly the most important thing to say about rheumatoid arthritis is that it is common and affects the emotional fabric of millions of people throughout the world. It is right at the top of the world's health problems along with cancer and heart disease, and is just as emotionally devastating. More importantly, it has been at that level of importance for many years and will remain there until research gives us a cause and, eventually, a cure.

We physicians often forget this most important emotional aspect of the disease as we calculate research dollars spent, lives disrupted, the cost of disability, and the overall impact such an illness has on society. We forget this most important aspect; namely, the toll which the disease takes on the person who has the unfortunate fate of getting rheumatoid arthritis, and on his or her loved ones.

Dr. Robert Phillips, in his book *Coping With Rheumatoid Arthritis*, has addressed the concerns of the RA patient and made the human side of this illness a priority. He is concerned with every aspect of how to "hang on," while we—the medical community—fumble for answers to one of the most important diseases of our age. Having RA, you have to learn to live or cope with an altered existence. You have to change your schedules, become "one" with your doctor or physical therapist, change your pace, and deal with such ordinary tasks as opening a jar or even driving a car. This book will help you appreciate life by helping you to understand a mystery. After reading this book you will value your life despite arthritis, and realize that overall you are still a lucky, living being who can think, savor emotion, and—with a strength of purpose—continue better than before.

As a doctor I learned more about my patients by reading this book. I will never look at the arthritic patient again without offering a borrowed phrase of encouragement from this book. Perhaps all physicians should learn to cope with patients who are learning to cope with this disease. I might even apply the tenets Dr. Phillips explains in my treatment and certainly my explanation of other diseases in the future.

Best of all, this book is almost all-encompassing. It is a work which will allow you, the patient, to confront science, understand your family's reactions to your illness, your financial concerns, your rational use of medicine, anger, pain, guilt, stress—the list goes on and on. If you are a relative or friend of an RA patient, you will live their struggle with empathy and understanding. You, too, will cope.

I would wish that all patients had access to the person of Dr. Phillips, but since that is not possible, you have the next best thing—his book. Read it, nod your head, agree with it, pass it on to your friends and those you cherish. It will enrich your life, their lives and, most of all, allow all of you to cope successfully with rheumatoid arthritis.

Robert G. Lahita, M.D., Ph.D.
Associate Professor
Hospital for Special Surgery
Cornell University
New York, NY

Preface

Rheumatoid arthritis can have quite an impact on you and your family. No kidding! Upon being diagnosed, many questions may come to mind. Physicians or other professionals may be able to answer some of them. Others may not have any answers, and this can be upsetting. It can also be upsetting to realize that this is happening to *you*. Discovering that you have rheumatoid arthritis can be very depressing.

Fortunately, medical science has made a great deal of progress in treating and controlling rheumatoid arthritis. So there is every chance that you will be able to lead a more normal and productive life. But what about the psychological effects of the disease? Will it interfere with your previous lifestyle? Will you be able to handle the pain? A major factor, then, in determining how normal and emotionally stable your life will be, is *how well you cope with rheumatoid arthritis*.

Powerful stuff? It certainly is, but now you know why this book was written in the first place! It's filled with facts, suggestions, techniques, strategies, and other useful ideas. It was written specifically for you and for members of your family and friends.

The first part of the book presents some background information about rheumatoid arthritis: what it is, what the symptoms are, an overview of how to treat it, and so on. The other sections deal with different aspects of living with the disease, including coping with emotions, changes in lifestyle, and living with others. These are all important aspects of coping with this or any other chronic condition. We will explore them in detail, and you'll find suggestions and strategies as well as illustrative examples for each component. In fact, a lot of the information you'll read can (and does!) apply to any chronic condition. In this book, however, the main focus is on your life with rheumatoid arthritis.

Remember that you are a unique person. Even though a lot of similarities exist, your own life with rheumatoid arthritis—the way it affects you and the way you experience it—will not be exactly the same as anyone else's. Therefore, it will be up to *you* to use the suggestions and strategies in this book to help you to cope as well as you possibly can. As you read about others' experiences, you'll see that you're not alone. Others feel the same way that you do, and this can be very reassuring.

Researchers are working hard, trying to find a cure for rheumatoid arthritis. But until that time, you'll have to learn to live with it. I hope this book is of help to you and your family. Remember: you can *always* improve the quality of your life.

Robert H. Phillips, Ph.D.
Center for Coping with Chronic Conditions
Long Island, NY

PART I.
Rheumatoid Arthritis—An Overview

1

Rheumatoid Arthritis— What Is It?

Marie, a 26-year-old mother of two, was in a lot of pain. In fact, she had been feeling achy and uncomfortable for quite a while now, and her pain just didn't seem to be going away. The pain was affecting her knees, hips, and shoulder joints, and it hurt to move. She felt like a "mummy," especially when she woke up in the morning. It seemed to take hours before she could move at all! Finally, her husband dragged her (painfully!) to the doctor, where she received a complete physical examination, a number of blood tests, and a series of x-rays. After analyzing all the results, the doctor gently sat Marie down and said, "You have rheumatoid arthritis." Marie's trembling reaction was, "I have *what*???"

Yes, Marie had rheumatoid arthritis (RA)—a chronic inflammatory disease primarily affecting the joints of the body. It is also referred to as a systemic disease because it can affect many other parts of the body. RA is a confusing, mystifying disease. It's puzzling because it is not completely understood. What causes it? What affects it? RA progresses differently in everyone. No two cases are ever exactly the same.

In order to better understand RA, let's talk a little bit about the main body part affected by this disease.

WELCOME TO THE JOINT!

"The ankle bone's connected to the shin bone; the shin bone's connected to the knee bone; the knee bone's connected to the thigh

3

bone . . ." and so on. You may recognize these lines as the lyrics to an old ditty which you've probably sung many times. But they're not anatomically correct! The bones are not directly connected to each other. Rather, they're connected by tendons, ligaments, and muscles. The area where the bones come together forms what we know as a joint (also called an articulation).

What's the joint for? It permits motion. So if you want to move your arm, walk, chew, or do a number of other things, your joints permit such activities.

The joint is a very important structure. Why? It's going to do a lot of hard work. Stop and think for a moment about the millions of times you move different joints in your body each day. Just today you've probably already yawned, snapped your fingers, stood up or sat down. In addition, every time you move, it's rarely one simple joint that's moving. Usually a number of joints are involved in any one movement. Think about how much wear and tear each of your joints will experience in your lifetime. It is remarkable to think that, for the most part, joint movement is smooth, frictionless, and pain-less.

TYPES OF JOINTS

All the joints in the skeleton can be grouped into three categories, depending on the kind and degree of movement they allow. The first category is the immovable joint. The joints of the skull would be one example. The bones of the skull fit together in an interlocking pattern to protect the brain.

The second type of joint is the slightly movable joint. Although the joints in this category do not move very much, there is a little bit of flexibility built into the joint structure. An example of this category would be the bones of the spinal column.

The third type of joint is the movable joint. Examples include the joints of the fingers, toes, hips, shoulders, and knees. These are the joints that may be primarily involved in rheumatoid arthritis. They are also the ones that are usually referred to in casual conversation on this topic.

Not all the joints are structured the same way. Nor is it necessary to go into detail concerning any of the other structures of the joint, such as the ligaments, the bursa, tendons, and muscles. Rather, this discussion should serve to emphasize the structures that are important in rheumatoid arthritis.

JOINT STRUCTURE AND FUNCTION

The space between the two bones meeting at a joint is called the joint space or cavity. The surrounding connective tissue enclosing this space is called the joint capsule. The joint capsule is actually composed of two layers. The outside layer is the thick, dense, tough, fibrous protective connective tissue. This tissue is fastened to each end of the bones forming the joint. Its purpose is to connect the bones and stabilize the joint.

The inside layer of the joint capsule is called the synovial membrane. This thin membrane protects the joint by removing small particles and debris from the joint cavity, and by producing a lubricating fluid called synovial fluid. The synovial fluid is a clear, pale yellow, slightly thickened, oily liquid. In rheumatoid arthritis, the synovial fluid is thinner than normal. Not only does this fluid lubricate the joint, but it also nourishes the cartilage, keeping it healthy (since the cartilage itself has no blood vessels).

Each joint capsule contains tiny blood vessels which nourish the joint structure. Even more important (especially to someone with rheumatoid arthritis) is the fact that nerves run through these capsules. These nerves conduct pain messages to the brain.

Problems that exist within the joint capsule may not be a matter of life or death. But if you have RA, they may mean the difference between comfort and pain.

CARTILAGE

Picture the ends of the two bones which meet at a joint. They need protection so they don't keep banging against each other, wearing each other out. So the end of each bone is covered by a smooth, white, connective tissue (up to an eighth of an inch thick) called cartilage. The structure of the cartilage creates smooth, elastic, resilient surfaces which can rub against each other with very little friction, especially when lubricated with the synovial fluid.

In normal cases, all parts of the joint (such as the bone, cartilage, and synovial fluid) work smoothly together. However, because there are so many parts, it's easy to understand how something can go wrong. That's where arthritic problems come in.

HOW DOES RA OCCUR?

In some cases, the onset of rheumatoid arthritis can be rapid and severe. But RA usually develops slowly. It may take months or even years. You may experience symptoms for a few days that will then disappear. They may reappear in a somewhat more severe form a little later on and then fade away once again. Often, when symptoms return, they seem to be stronger than before.

The return of symptoms (flares or exacerbations) alternates with the disappearance or decrease of symptoms (remissions). These cycles are typical of rheumatoid arthritis. Days, weeks, or months may go by between flares or remissions, but it is impossible to predict how long any particular phase will last. Unfortunately, in some cases the disease may remain in a flare for longer and longer periods until remissions seem virtually nonexistent.

Rheumatoid arthritis can range from extremely mild to quite severe. With mild RA you may notice only passing pain, sporadic swelling, or some stiffness in your joints. This may not last too long. It can be uncomfortable but usually doesn't lead to seriously-deformed joints. You may not even bother to contact a doctor. (In general, however, it's a good idea to obtain ongoing medical treatment to make sure the symptoms do not indicate permanent damage.)

With more severe RA, other things may occur. RA can cause your joints to become painful, swollen, warm, tender, or stiff. (These are the basic symptoms of inflammation in the joint). Continued inflammation can sometimes cause the joint to become deformed, disfigured or crippled.

Rheumatoid arthritis seems to affect certain joints more than others. For example, each of your fingers has three joints: the base, the middle, and the tip. Rheumatoid arthritis is much more likely to affect the base and middle joint than the tip joint. It's also more likely to affect the joints at the base of your toes.

Rheumatoid arthritis usually affects several joints. It rarely affects just one. The joints most often involved are the knees, hands, wrists, and feet. Usually, joints on both sides of the body become affected, such as both hands, both wrists, or both shoulders. This is referred to as "being symmetrical," and is characteristic of RA. But in some cases, only a few joints may be involved in a non-symmetrical manner. This may lead to a delay in diagnosis because it is an unusual case.

Symptoms of RA

Symptoms vary from person to person. They can even vary within the same person from time to time. The symptoms can come and go, often very quickly and without warning.

What are the first symptoms of RA? Usually fatigue, stiffness, soreness, change of appetite, weight loss, as well as aching sensations. You may experience stiffness in your muscles early in the morning, or after you sit or stand still for a long period of time. Frequently this stiffness will ease up after you get up and move around for a while, or after a warm shower or bath.

When do the first symptoms tend to occur? It's hard to say what, exactly, causes the first onset of symptoms. Some people feel that it may come after a physiologically stressful situation which affects the body, such as an acute infection or injury. But there is no definitive proof of this. Others feel that emotional stress may be the precipitator, such as the death of a loved one, separation or divorce. Some people feel that other types of emotional problems, such as difficulty at work or within the family, can trigger an attack of RA. It is important to remember, however, that *most of the time there is no specific factor that can be pinpointed.*

In addition to the symptoms mentioned previously, others do occasionally occur. In some cases, inflammation in and around the joint can damage other tissues drastically, especially the tendons. Tendon rupture may occur, leaving the bones unable to move or function properly.

People with RA often have anemia, especially if their case of RA is severe. You may develop rheumatoid nodules, which are little lumps that grow under the skin. Your lymph nodes may enlarge. Some people may experience eye problems because of RA.

With particularly severe RA, inflammation may affect your blood vessels (vasculitis), the sac surrounding your heart (pericarditis), the lining of your lungs (pleuritis), or the lining of your eyes (scleritis), among other areas. RA can affect virtually any system of your body.

Let's Talk About Inflammation

Rheumatoid arthritis is a chronic inflammatory disease. Therefore, it makes sense that the major problem in rheumatoid arthritis would be inflammation! Normally, inflammation isn't really a bad thing. It is the body's way of protecting itself, controlling infection, and repairing injuries. In most cases, once any damage has been repaired, inflammation subsides. But in the case of rheumatoid arthritis, something goes wrong with the inflammation process and it becomes destructive. It gets out of control. The synovial membrane, the tissue lining the joint capsule, becomes inflamed. This inflammation causes the joint lining to thicken, swell, and spread out, covering the surface of the joint. It then ends up causing even more tissue damage instead of repairing the tissue.

Inflammation causes your joint to appear swollen, and it feels puffy when touched. Inflammation leads to increased blood flow. That's what makes the joint feel warm and appear red. Another part of the inflammation process is the release of enzymes from the white blood cells and synovial membrane cells in the joint. These enzymes cause further irritation, continuing the inflammation process. They also produce pain.

Pain results from excess fluid (due to the swelling) distending the joint capsule where there are pressure-sensitive nerve endings. Pain is also caused by the irritating chemicals which are produced by the white blood cells and inflamed synovial membrane cells. Finally, some pain occurs as a result of weakened muscles and spasms in muscles surrounding the inflamed joint.

In rheumatoid arthritis, the inflammatory white blood cells enter the synovial membrane. There is a tremendous increase in the number of synovial membrane cells, an increase in capillaries inside the synovial membrane, and also an increase in connective tissue within the synovial membrane. The once-thin membrane now becomes quite thick, and is called a pannus.

The inflammatory pannus can stretch and damage the other supportive connective tissues, such as the tendons and ligaments. This weakens the joints, making them unstable and leading to possible dislocations and deformities. Movement is reduced—and hurts! In addition, the inflammation interferes with the smooth, frictionless, pain-free operation of the joint. This is a common feature of RA.

WHO GETS RA?

If you have rheumatoid arthritis, you are in the company of such famous historical figures as Christopher Columbus, President James Madison, Renoir (the French painter), and Mary Queen of Scots! Other famous people have rheumatoid arthritis, too, but this is a book of coping—not of stargazing!

RA is a common disease. It is estimated that five to seven million people in the United States alone have rheumatoid arthritis. Approximately 75% of those with RA are women. RA can begin at virtually any age—from infancy to old age—but is most commonly noticed between the ages of thirty and sixty.

All in the Family?

A few studies suggest that there may be a family history of rheumatoid arthritis. Other studies state that, although there may be a genetic link to the illness, most people with RA have no family history of RA and will not pass it on to their children.

Where Does RA Occur?

Although people feel that different types of regions may have a higher incidence of RA, there is no specific geographic location that is more or less prone to rheumatoid arthritis. It seems that individuals in all parts of the world can develop RA. Climate also seems to be of little importance. You might prefer a certain type of climate, but research has not yet proven that any type of climate plays a significant role in the development or progression of rheumatoid arthritis.

What *does* play a significant role? Good question—one that will be discussed in Chapter 2!

2

Causes Of Rheumatoid Arthritis

The underlying cause of rheumatoid arthritis is still a mystery, although a lot of researchers are trying to find the answer.

What are the most probable theories? The first is the infection theory. Some scientists believe that rheumatoid arthritis is caused by some type of foreign substance or microorganism, such as a virus, which causes an infection. Perhaps a virus can trigger the onset of rheumatoid arthritis in people who have a genetic predisposition to the disease. Maybe this virus triggers the inflammatory process which exacerbates rheumatoid arthritis. So far, scientists haven't been able to isolate it. Since there isn't too much evidence yet available, this remains a questionable—although possible—theory.

The second theory centers around the idea that something is confusing your immune system. Maybe your body is having difficulty distinguishing foreign invaders from your own tissues, so your immune system begins fighting healthy tissues. This reaction can also be called an "auto-immune response." In other words, there is a "defense mechanism reaction" or an allergy to your own tissue.

The third, and most recent, theory is actually a combination of the first two. The rheumatoid factor found in the bloodstream of many people with RA also seems to appear in individuals (as well as laboratory animals) with chronic infections. It seems to disappear once the infection is cured. This tends to support a combination of the two theories. Why? If you get an infection in your body, this may stimulate your immune system. This may lead to the production of rheumatoid factor, a type of antibody (more about this in a minute) which participates in creating the inflammatory response within the joint.

Foreign invaders that cause the immune system to respond are called antigens. When an antigen is present in the body, it usually stimulates the production of antibodies. These antibodies are developed in order to fight and conquer the antigens. The problem with rheumatoid arthritis is that it causes the body's immune system to turn against itself. The most frequent site of this reaction is the joint. In addition, in more complicated cases, the lungs, blood vessels, heart, and other tissues are attacked as if they were antigens or foreign invaders.

ANY OTHER THOUGHTS?

Is stress a cause of rheumatoid arthritis? Research has suggested that, for the most part, it isn't. More widely accepted is the fact that stress can exacerbate an existing condition. But regardless of the cause of RA, once it has been diagnosed, the important issue is how it's treated. The next chapter will review ways in which RA is diagnosed; then we'll move on to its treatment.

3

Diagnosing Rheumatoid Arthritis

Remember Marie from Chapter 1? She knew she was in pain, but couldn't believe she had rheumatoid arthritis. So she asked her doctor how the diagnosis was made. She learned that RA is not the easiest disease to diagnose. Let's talk about why.

To come up with a correct diagnosis of RA, a physician may need to observe you for awhile. Although RA may be suspected, a definitive diagnosis takes time—sometimes up to several months. It may be necessary for you to visit your physician several times before a confirmed diagnosis is possible. This is because there is no one specific test that offers positive proof that you have RA. It may be necessary to gather a good deal of information before a physician can be sure of the diagnosis.

In order for your doctor to accurately diagnose RA, any of a number of methods may be necessary, including a complete medical history, physical examination, blood and laboratory tests, and x-rays, among others. Current symptoms and a physical examination are the most important parts of the diagnostic procedure. Laboratory tests may be useful as additional evidence that the physician's diagnosis is correct.

MEDICAL HISTORY

The first step is for your doctor to receive a detailed medical history from you. What are some of the more important questions? "Where are the aches and pains?" "What joints hurt?" "How long have they hurt?" (One of the first requirements for diagnosis is for you to have experienced pain and swelling in one or more joints for at least six weeks.) "What seems to help them?" "What time of day do they bother you the most?" "Do the joints feel warm and swollen; do they look red?" "What injuries may have caused the inflammation?" "Do you experience any fever, chills, or weight changes?" "Do you feel more tired or fatigued than usual?" These are among the many questions that may be asked.

PHYSICAL EXAMINATION

During the physical exam, the physician tries to determine your general state of health, as well as what specific symptoms exist. Your physician will check your joints carefully. He will look, touch, and listen for any kind of abnormality.

Your physician will carefully examine any joints that seem to be abnormal: joints that show signs of tenderness, redness, warmth, swelling, or inflammation. Physicians will also carefully observe you as you attempt to move certain joints, looking for any signs of pain or reduced movement. The doctor will check your muscles for any signs of weakness or spasm. Finally, he'll check you for signs of rheumatoid arthritis not involving the joints: nodules under the skin (especially by the elbows), dryness of the eyes or mouth, inflamed eyes, lung inflammation or pleurisy, rashes, and so forth.

LABORATORY TESTS

There are many laboratory tests available, but none of them are definitive in diagnosing RA. Similar lab tests come out positive for many different forms of arthritis, especially in the early stages.

Blood Tests

A complete blood count is one test which may be helpful. This provides a count of the many different types of blood cells in your body. Hemoglobin tests and the hematocrit are used to assess the red blood cells. A low number of red blood cells, indicating anemia, is common in individuals who have chronic inflammation as a result of rheumatoid arthritis.

Testing the blood for the number of white blood cells and evaluating the different types of white cells is also important. Because white blood cells are essential to fighting infection, the number of white blood cells is usually increased in RA. Sometimes, however, the number of white blood cells is decreased. One reason for this might be a reaction to certain medication.

Another blood test is the erythrocyte sedimentation rate (ESR). This test measures the distance that red blood cells settle toward the bottom of a narrow tube in one hour. If the blood cells settle more quickly (in other words, the blood cells fall many millimeters), it is said that the ESR or "sed rate" is high. Individuals who experience inflammation because of RA tend to have a high sed rate. The rate of sedimentation (settling) increases if your body has chronic inflammation. As you get better (as RA improves), the sed rate usually becomes lower. The ESR can also be high due to anemia and the presence of a lot of antibodies in the blood.

The sed rate test doesn't necessarily help in diagnosis. So why is it used? It can help to determine how serious your RA may be. The higher the sed rate, the more inflammation that exists. This may mean that your disease is more active. By following the sed rate over a period of time, your doctor may learn whether the amount of inflammation is increasing or decreasing.

One of the more common tests for people with RA is the test for rheumatoid factor. One method of testing for rheumatoid factor antibodies is the latex test. This test measures whether or not the rheumatoid factor is present in your blood and, if so, just how much rheumatoid factor is present (the titer). Most people with RA have high amounts of rheumatoid factor in their blood. However, it is estimated that 20% of individuals with RA do not have rheumatoid factor antibodies. Another problem is that people other than those with RA have rheumatoid factor. It may be found in individuals with other diseases, and even in healthy people. If your latex test is positive, does this mean you definitely have rheumatoid arthritis? Not necessarily, but it's certainly a piece of supportive evidence. Although 80% of people with RA eventually test positive in a latex test for rheumatoid factor, it may come out negative in the early months of the disease in an even higher percentage of people.

Another antibody which may be found in some people with RA (although it's more commonly seen in illnesses such as scleroderma and lupus) is the antinuclear antibody. The ANA test is used to determine its presence. Estimates say that 25% of those with RA have this antibody in their blood.

Joint Aspiration (Arthrocentesis)

Sometimes a doctor will remove some synovial fluid from your joint using a special kind of hypodermic syringe. This is called joint aspiration. Doctors examine the fluid to see if they can learn what's causing your inflammation. They may test the fluid for white blood cells, bacteria, rheumatoid factor, or other things.

The joint aspiration test is pretty easy, especially when it is done in the knee. It doesn't have to be done in the hospital and there are very few complications (the most common of which is infection).

Biopsies

In some instances, when the reason for joint swelling is still not understood, a physician may decide to remove a little piece of tissue from the synovial membrane. This tissue is then examined under the microscope by a pathologist. On occasion, a biopsy may be taken from a skin rash area, muscle, nodule under the skin, or other location if the microscope findings can be helpful in planning the most productive treatment.

Arthroscopy

Doctors can also use a device—similar to a miniature telescope—to look directly inside a joint. This comparatively new procedure is known as arthroscopy. Because the procedure is an invasive one (meaning that it goes inside your body), it's done in an operating room. It's usually performed under general anesthesia, but can sometimes be done under local anesthesia. The tiny arthroscope is inserted into the joint. The doctor then inspects the tissues of the joint. It's important to examine the cartilage for possible damage. If any injury is found that is treatable, the surgeon can sometimes repair it through another tiny entry hole made next to it. Otherwise, the arthroscope is used mainly for diagnostic purposes.

X-Rays

X-rays can be an important part of diagnosing RA. However, they are primarily useful only when the disease has advanced to the stage where they can actually *show* something. Earlier on, x-rays may not clearly show damage to the bones or cartilage. However, there's still an advantage to early x-rays. They provide a baseline, against which later x-rays can be compared to see how the disease is advancing or if the illness is causing further deterioration. They are also an indication to doctors as to how well treatment programs are controlling the progression of the disease. X-rays can also identify where sufficient bone damage exists to necessitate joint replacement surgery.

4

Treatment Of Rheumatoid Arthritis

As soon as Marie understood how her RA was diagnosed, her next question wasn't surprising. "What can you do to treat my condition?" This is the most important question for most people with RA.

Some unhappy people believe that, once you have RA, you can't do much to stop it from progressing into a severely crippling, deforming and incapacitating illness. This couldn't be further from the truth. Sure, there are a few cases where RA may continue to progress despite all therapeutic efforts. However, in most cases a good, comprehensive treatment program can help you to live a comfortable and satisfying (if not totally pain-free) life.

How do you determine the best treatment for your RA? Unfortunately, this is usually a trial-and-error process. But you can help—by understanding the disease and the way it works, and by carefully following your treatment program.

GOALS OF TREATMENT

Why is treatment of RA so frustrating? One reason is because there's no magic cure. There's no pill that will make RA go away. There's no surgical procedure that will eliminate the illness. There's no injection that will restore a joint to its original healthy condition. No treatment is 100% effective in controlling *all* symptoms. Since RA cannot be fully cured, it's better to consider your treatment program as more of a management program. But treatment for RA *can* be very positive and productive.

What is the most important goal of treatment? To help you to live as normal a life as possible. Treatments (such as pain killers) that attempt to instantly alleviate certain symptoms may not be right for you. Why? They may help you to feel better at the moment, but may not do anything to stop the disease from progressing.

Hopefully, treatment for RA will bring about an extended or even permanent remission. Although this may not always be possible, it's certainly a goal worth shooting for. There's no way to predict whether or not it can happen in your case but, in general, treatment programs have been becoming more and more effective. If remission is not possible, at least you'll aim to suppress symptoms, helping you to live with the disease more effectively and comfortably.

What are the general goals of treatment? There are basically five: (1) To reduce or relieve pain, (2) To reduce inflammation, (3) To preserve function, (4) To maintain or increase strength and mobility, allowing you to keep your joints functioning as smoothly and as effectively as possible, and (5) To prevent deformity. If your joints have already been damaged, your treatment program will aim to prevent further damage, and to avoid deformities. Additional treatment may attempt to correct any deformities that have already occurred.

WHO PLANS YOUR TREATMENT?

Treatment programs are usually developed by a team of health care professionals, including physicians, physical therapists, occupational therapists, social workers, and rehab specialists. Initially, your physician may be the most directly involved in planning your treatment program.

COMPONENTS OF TREATMENT PROGRAMS

Because there is no one particular treatment that is best for every person with RA, the program that you'll follow is a "package"—a combination of modalities.

Your treatment program may include any—or all—of the following: rest, exercise, medication (to control pain and reduce inflammation), physical aids and other assistance devices, physical therapy, and other methods to control pain and improve mobility. Occasionally, surgery may be an adjunct to the treatment program. Any complete treatment program also attempts to help you deal with the emotional difficulties you may experience as a result of your RA—not just the physical difficulties.

Finally, and very importantly, treatment programs include a modified and improved long-term change in lifestyle. More detail regarding these components will be found in Part III, *Changes In General Lifestyle*.

WHAT TREATMENT IS BEST?

Because RA can affect different people in different ways, each treatment program is individual and unique. Your own treatment program will vary, and depends on many factors. For example, how severe is your RA? How long have you had it? Which joints are affected? Are any other systems of your body affected? Other factors such as your age, overall general health, family situation, lifestyle, and occupation are also taken into consideration.

Most treatment programs take a sensible, conservative approach. Physicians believe that this is best for long-term progress and results. This is usually better than a very aggressive program that expects immediate, spectacular results.

WHAT'S THE PROGNOSIS?

What is the prognosis for rheumatoid arthritis? Doctors have a difficult time predicting how it will affect any particular individual. Estimates are that 75% of the individuals who begin treatment for RA early in the course of the disease will improve significantly. Some may go into remission, with no current symptoms.

Other than your conscientious involvement, what's the most critical variable? Proper treatment! Without it, rheumatoid arthritis can be a progressive disease. It's possible that it can progress to the point where serious deformities and disabilities will occur. And, unfortunately, any bone or joint damage that occurs is irreversible. Bone damage doesn't go away.

Who has a more difficult time with RA? If you've had chronic persistent rheumatoid arthritis for more than a year, if your rheumatoid arthritis began before the age of thirty, if you have rheumatoid nodules under your skin, or if you have high amounts of the rheumatoid factor, you may experience more difficulty with RA. However, with proper treatment the prognosis can *still* be favorable. For example, it is estimated that only one in six individuals with rheumatoid arthritis develops severe enough symptoms to result in any deformity or crippling. In all probability, even these could have been prevented with early, effective treatment. If properly treated, even the worst cases of rheumatoid arthritis can get better over a period of time. The disease itself can become less aggressive. The inflammation can become less active. Other symptoms can decrease in intensity. Most people with rheumatoid arthritis can be prevented from experiencing serious trouble and can continue to live satisfying, productive lives.

Additional improvements are expected in the future with new drugs and additional surgical procedures which can restore comfort and mobility to affected joints.

Despite all this, RA is still considered a major national health problem. Why? It is very common and quite painful. It can damage your joints and can disrupt your life. But, remember, it is possible for you to learn to come to grips with the discomforts of rheumatoid arthritis.

Learn about your illness. If you learn about RA, you can fight it better. Reading books, attending courses and seminars, among other activities, will help you to gain knowledge of RA. All these activities are offered by The Arthritis Foundation. Don't be afraid to ask your doctor any questions you may have. If you are informed and educated, you'll even be able to assist your doctor in your care.

You can help your prognosis! Make sure you seek prompt medical attention. Make sure you properly comply with your prescribed treatment!

Treatment results will be slow in coming. Don't expect overnight success. However, with patience and proper adherence to a treatment program, you *can* experience significant improvement!

5

Juvenile Rheumatoid Arthritis

It's sad to see children suffering from the pain of arthritis. There may be many different forms of arthritis in youngsters. The most common, by far, is juvenile rheumatoid arthritis (JRA). This disease is also known as juvenile arthritis, Still's disease, or juvenile chronic polyarthritis.

JRA usually strikes before the child reaches the age of sixteen. In rare cases, it occurs as early as six weeks of age. Most commonly, it occurs between the ages of two and five and nine and twelve. It is more likely for girls to be affected by the illness than boys.

As in rheumatoid arthritis, the major symptom in JRA is inflammation. The synovial membrane that lines the joint swells and overgrows. The joint becomes stiff and painful with swelling, warmth, and sometimes redness of the skin over the involved joint.

Long-lasting inflammation, especially in children with severe JRA, can damage surfaces of the joint. If this happens, the joint damage may lead to the types of deformities that are noticeable in adults with RA. Fortunately, this doesn't happen very often.

A problem that children with JRA have is that inflammation of the joints may affect bone growth. It is estimated that approximately half of the individuals affected by JRA experience a disturbance of growth patterns and development while the disease is active. If this occurs for a long period of time, the child's overall physical development may be slowed. However, when JRA is in remission, or if treatment and proper medical care have it under control, growth resumes and normal development is possible.

SYMPTOMS

As with adult RA, JRA has a great variety of symptoms and complications. General symptoms and signs of JRA can change from one day to the next—even from hour to hour. Pain and stiffness in the joints may be mild one day, but so severe the next day that the child is unable to move without a great deal of discomfort.

JRA has been called the "hidden handicap." The reason for this is that most of the pain and damage that occurs is inside and isn't obvious to others. However, slowed growth (shorter height), joint damage, stiff walking, or deformity in fingers or wrists may make it more noticeable.

THE THREE TYPES OF JRA

Until recently, doctors believed that JRA was one single chronic disease. However, it is now recognized that there are at least three different forms of JRA. Inflammation is a common component of all three types of JRA, but each may begin in a different way. So although there are similarities, JRA is not exactly the same as the adult form of RA.

The first form is called systemic JRA. This can affect many different areas of the body, including internal organs and systems. The second form is called polyarticular JRA. "Poly" means "several" or "many," and "articular" means "joint." Therefore, polyarticular JRA can affect many different joints. The third type is called pauciarticular JRA. "Pauc" means "few," so pauciarticular JRA affects only a few joints.

Let's talk about these three forms of JRA in a little more detail.

Systemic JRA

This is the type of JRA that is often referred to as Still's disease. Systemic JRA usually affects boys and girls to a comparable degree. Children of any age can be affected, and it is estimated that approximately 20% of all cases of JRA fall into this category. It is unusual for this type of RA to occur in similar form in adults, although it sometimes does.

High fever is frequently a symptom of systemic JRA. The fever may begin in the evening and can go up to 103° or higher. Within a few hours, the temperature will probably return to normal, only to rebound the next day. On occasion, two fever spikes may occur in a single day. The high fever is usually accompanied by chills and may cause the child to feel very sick. These fluctuating fevers can last for weeks or even months, but usually never longer than six months (at the very worst).

A rash is another common symptom that may accompany fever (or it may exist on its own). Similar to the ups and downs of the fever, the rash may come and go for several hours or days. It may appear only briefly, possibly when the temperature is high. It may also occur following a shower or hot bath. The rash usually appears as pale red spots on the chest or thighs. It may occasionally be present on other parts of the body as well. Although rashes aren't very pleasant, they can help physicians to diagnose JRA. This can help treatment to begin as early as possible.

Systemic JRA can affect many joints. Joint involvement may begin at the same time as the fevers or long after. Some children experience pain in the joints only during a fever, and feel better once their temperature goes down. On occasion, joint problems may remain a long-lasting problem for children with systemic JRA.

Joint pain may exist to some degree, a minimal degree, or not at all. Pain may occur periodically, lasting for days or weeks, or disappearing as suddenly as it began.

Systemic JRA may also affect the outer lining of the heart (pericarditis) or the lungs (pleuritis). There may also be an enlargement of the lymph nodes and occasionally the liver and spleen. Other organs may be involved as well. Systemic JRA may lead to severe anemia, and can cause stomach pain.

Children with systemic JRA need to be monitored carefully and require regular doctor visits. In this way, treatment can be as effective and specific as possible. On occasion, if the illness becomes severe enough, the child may require hospitalization.

Polyarticular JRA

According to estimates, approximately 40-50% of all children who develop JRA have the polyarticular form. Polyarticular JRA tends to develop more in girls than in boys.

By definition, polyarticular JRA affects five or more joints. Which joints are affected? Polyarticular JRA usually appears in the small joints of the fingers and hands (such as the knuckles and wrists) and occasionally in weight-bearing joints such as the hips, knees, ankles, and feet. Polyarticular JRA is often symmetrical. Slight fever occasionally occurs in some children.

The main characteristic of polyarticular JRA is intense inflammation of the synovial membrane. Because polyarticular JRA is often identical to adult RA, it is possible that polyarticular JRA (more than the other forms of JRA) can last until adulthood. Rheumatoid factor may be present in the blood of some children with this form of JRA. Rheumatoid nodules on the elbows or other parts of the body are most likely to develop in this type of JRA.

Pauciarticular JRA

Estimates are that 30-40% of children with JRA have the pauciarticular form. By definition, pauciarticular JRA affects four or fewer joints. The joints that are usually involved are the large joints such as the knees, elbows, or ankles. Pauciarticular JRA is usually not symmetrical. Most children with pauciarticular arthritis feel fine overall, except for pain or stiffness in the affected joints.

A subcategory of pauciarticular JRA would be monoarticular JRA. This simply means that the disease affects only one joint. In children, this joint is usually the knee.

Boys with pauciarticular JRA are more likely to experience stiffness in their hips. Lower back stiffness is a common symptom early in the disease. Other large joints may be affected. It's not unusual for boys who develop this type of pauciarticular JRA to develop ankylosing spondylitis—an inflammatory disease of the spine.

Children with pauciarticular JRA are at a higher risk of developing eye inflammation. This causes eye pain and red eyes, and can affect vision. Because of this, it's important to have frequent eye examinations. In this way, treatment for eye problems can hopefully prevent any vision loss.

CAUSES OF JRA

As with adult RA, it is not known what causes JRA. Because JRA rarely occurs in more than one child per family, it doesn't seem to be a hereditary illness. So if there *is* a genetic predisposition to JRA, this certainly isn't the only cause.

DIAGNOSING JRA

It's difficult to diagnose JRA. Why? Because there are so many different symptoms, there are three different forms of JRA, and signs and symptoms can vary from child to child.

Diagnosing JRA is similar to diagnosing adult RA. In both, a medical history, physical examination, laboratory tests, and x-rays may be used. On occasion, joint tissue or fluid will be examined.

JRA is usually not diagnosed unless symptoms have existed for at least six consecutive weeks. This may be a problem, since some children are not as aware of pain as others. They may not even report pain when JRA does exist. In such cases, a clue for JRA could be a limp or some other sign that the child is experiencing difficulties, such as not being able to move the neck to look up.

Physicians will look for some evidence of joint inflammation. If a child complains of aches and pains, but doesn't show changes in the joints or evidence of inflammation, JRA may not be the correct diagnosis. However, in systemic JRA, joint involvement may be hard to detect early in the disease.

What else will doctors look for in trying to diagnose JRA? They'll look for the rash that is common in systemic JRA, the rheumatoid nodules that can occur in polyarticular JRA, or even the eye problems that may occur in pauciarticular JRA.

X-rays of the joints may be helpful, although not specifically for diagnosing JRA. At least they can determine the structure of the joints. As with adult RA, they may also be useful as a basis for comparison with future x-rays.

The whole diagnostic procedure can be very frustrating for the child and especially for the parents. There are a lot of uncertainties involved, and a long period of time can elapse before a definitive diagnosis is reached.

TREATING JRA

Principles of management and treatment of juvenile rheumatoid arthritis are similar to those in adult rheumatoid arthritis. The first step in treating JRA is to receive an accurate diagnosis (of course). Treatment programs usually include rest, exercise, medication, a balanced diet, and eye care. If long-term problems exist, other types of treatment (such as surgery) may be necessary. A proper and aggressive treatment program is important in order to prevent the possibility of joint deformity. As with adult RA, treatment programs will be modified as needed. Unfortunately, however, there is no rapid solution to JRA.

Specific treatment for JRA depends on who has it. Boy or girl? Age? Severity of the disease? Type of JRA? Symptoms involved? Parts of the body affected?

PROGNOSIS

Although JRA is considered a chronic disease, the long-term outlook is good. Many children who develop it will see symptoms disappear as they grow into adulthood and will experience little or no permanent disability as a result of the disease. It is estimated that approximately 75% of all children with JRA will have normal joint function, or nearly normal joint function, by the time they reach adulthood. In some cases, however, there may be more serious complications. Eye problems can result from JRA. The best way to conquer such problems is to "prevent" them with early diagnosis and treatment. The prognosis is much better for Still's disease and for pauciarticular RA that it is for polyarticular JRA. Why? The latter is most similar to adult RA, and may continue into adulthood. The older the child is at the onset, the more likely that the condition will persist into adulthood. Young children's disease often disappears during adolescence.

In general, a child with JRA who receives prompt, effective medical treatment—along with the care, love, and warmth of family support—has a good chance of a complete recovery. The prognosis for children with JRA seems to be better than for adults with RA.

COPING WITH JRA

This condition can be as difficult to cope with as any other. Parents may have a hard time dealing with JRA because their child seems to be suffering continuously. It can be reassuring to know that children with JRA seem to do well in the long run.

It's important for parents to recognize that the child with JRA has good days and bad days. Emotional manifestations during bad times need to be understood and supported. On the other hand, it's important not to smother or pamper your child *too* much.

It's usually possible for children with JRA to keep up with school, social and other commitments. There may be short periods of time when changes in schedule may be necessary if the disease is in a severe stage or if joints have been damaged by the disease. However, if treatment remains effective, it is possible for most children with JRA to live fairly normal lives.

Much of the information provided in the rest of this book is suitable for those of you who live with JRA as well as adult RA. (And be sure you don't miss the chapters on the child and adolescent with JRA, in Part V.)

PART II.
Your Emotions

6

Coping With Your Emotions—An Introduction

How happy are you about having RA? Well, each person's emotional responses to RA are different. Even your own reactions to RA will vary from time to time. The more severe your reactions are, the more these will interfere with your ability to cope.

Your emotional reactions to RA may start even before treatment has begun. Of course, your reaction will also depend on how suddenly your condition developed. For example, if your condition developed very slowly, taking months or even years, you might adjust well, since you've had plenty of time to prepare.

When first diagnosed, some people may not even react, since it still may not be "real" to them. But others go through a hard time. You may know someone who has RA, or have heard about the experiences of some people with RA. Perhaps this frightened you. Emotional reactions to RA are not always rational. As a matter of fact, in many cases they are completely irrational. As the full impact of the diagnosis sets in, you may experience a whole variety of emotional reactions, ranging from sadness and anxiety to anger, frustration, and despair.

FACTORS SHAPING YOUR EMOTIONAL REACTIONS

Several factors may play a role in determining how you react to RA. Keep in mind, however, that because there are so many factors, no one can predict how a person will react at any given time. How did you handle problems before your condition was diagnosed? What was your general coping style? Were you calm or nervous? Were you persistent or did you give up easily? The way you handle life's problems in general will indicate how well you will cope with RA and its treatment. Are you successful in coping with stress? Stress in RA is related partly to how fast your condition developed and what kind of treatment you'll need, among other factors. Your age has a bearing on how you respond emotionally. Your general physical health prior to the onset of RA also plays a role in determining your coping ability. And what about your relationships? In many cases, your emotional reactions may reflect the responses of significant other people in your life. For example, if family members or friends are anxious about your medical condition, this may affect your emotional reactions.

WHICH EMOTIONAL REACTIONS?

Do you like yourself less since your diagnosis? Previous feelings of confidence can be quickly shattered. This loss of self-esteem can have a very unpleasant effect on you. You may not feel or behave like yourself. You'll want to deal with this right away in order to return to effective, efficient functioning.

Have you felt intense anger because you have to go through all this? Are you angry that your life will change because of RA? Are you afraid of the medication you may need? Do you become depressed when you compare your present life to the way things were? Have you felt afraid of not being able to cope? Do you fear facing a bleak, if not hopeless, future? Some of the most common emotional reactions to RA are depression, fear, guilt, and anger. Because of the importance of coping with these emotions, a separate chapter has been devoted to each of them.

MANAGING EMOTIONAL REACTIONS

Some of the ways people have adjusted to RA and its treatment have included therapeutic intervention, support groups, and education. Because your emotions play such an important role in life with RA, you'll certainly want to do the best possible job controlling them. How? Let's discuss some of the more important ways.

Medical Management

Make sure you're getting the best possible medical care. If you haven't already done so, you'll want to establish a good working relationship with your physician. This involves seeing a doctor who not only has expertise in treating RA but is also understanding and sympathetic to your emotional needs. You'll want to be sure that your physician watches your condition carefully, so any problems that may arise can be caught early. Your physician must also monitor your doses of medication carefully, so that they are used most effectively and any side effects are minimized.

Support Groups

Self-help or support groups can be very helpful. You'll see how others handle problems, some of which may be the same as, or at least similar to, your own. Groups provide a forum for the exchange of feelings and ideas, as well as suggestions on how to cope better. You'll see that you're not alone. This is probably the most important reason for belonging to a group. These groups are also wonderful for your family, giving members the chance to get some support of their own. Since one of the best ways to be in control of your emotions is to have a supportive family behind you, you should encourage their participation, too.

Do you ever feel shunned or ignored by others (or do you fear feeling this way)? Are your social relationships dwindling? Groups can give you a feeling of belonging. There are people that you can be with—people who share a common bond—because they, too, are living with RA.

In groups, any topics you'd like to talk about can be discussed. You may begin to share feelings more openly when you hear others talking about subjects you were previously reluctant to bring up yourself. As a result, a feeling of closeness (almost like family) develops.

Belonging to a national organization, such as the Arthritis Foundation, can be helpful. Such organizations bring patients and families together, and provide lots of beneficial information. They also help to expand public awareness about RA and its treatment. This will also help you with your emotions, since the more people who understand what's involved with RA, the less alone and isolated you'll feel.

By the way, there's no law that says that emotional reactions *have* to be shared with others. It's not necessary to talk them out, even though this can be helpful. But these emotional reactions do need to be recognized and worked through. That's the only way to make progress.

Medication

You'll frequently hear about medications that improve depression, anxiety, anger, and other emotional problems. Medication prescribed for these purposes is usually not addictive, so you might not be as reluctant to take it. Antianxiety medication can be helpful. So can mood elevators and antidepressants. But just remember that your doctor is the one who is in charge of medication. Don't "play with fire."

Psychological Strategies

Professional intervention may be necessary if your emotional problems are severe, or if you want to prevent them from getting worse. Having somebody to talk to can be a big help, especially with an illness like RA that has its ups and downs.

HELPING YOURSELF

Let's discuss some of the best techniques you can use to improve the way you feel.

Laugh a Little

Humor can be an amusingly effective way to deal with emotions. Whether it is hearing a joke from someone else, laughing at yourself, or creating your own jokes, humor can be a very relaxing way of dealing with a troublesome situation.

Humor works in three ways. First of all, it reduces anxiety. Laughing is a great way to release tension. Second, it can distract you from those things or feelings that are bothering you. When you're involved in something humorous, you often feel a lot better. Think back, for example, to a time when you were depressed or uncomfortable and somebody asked if you had heard a certain joke. Initially you may have been reluctant to hear it. But before long you were probably totally absorbed in the joke, wondering what the punch line would be! The fact that humor can distract you also means that it can help you to see things from a different perspective. So you may be able to look at something more objectively, which can help you to handle it more effectively.

Finally, the ability to laugh at yourself is a helpful coping strategy. It's also an important part of maturing. How well this works, however, depends on what you're going through. It's just about impossible (and probably ridiculous) to laugh at yourself while you're going through a crisis. However, as you adjust to your condition, you can better use humor as a coping strategy.

Relaxation Procedures

Relaxation is the opposite of tension. So if you learn to relax, you'll be much less tense. But relaxation procedures, by themselves, will not totally control your emotions. So why use them? Because if you're feeling more relaxed, you'll be better able to identify those problems that are affecting you, and you'll then be better able to figure out how to deal with them. Relaxation procedures, then, can be an essential first step in coping with your emotions.

How do you relax? We're talking about clinical relaxation, now—not everyday activities like reading, gardening, listening to music, or sitting in front of the television with a can of beer! There are different types of clinical relaxation procedures. For example, *progressive relaxation* is a procedure in which you learn how to relax the muscles in your body. *Hypnosis* is another relaxation procedure, as is meditation and *the relaxation response*. There's also a procedure called *imagery*, in which you view pictures in your mind that will help to relax you, thereby making it easier for you to solve problems. (More information about imagery can be found in the later chapter on Pain.) Books on any of these procedures are available in your local library, and can really help you to start feeling better.

Here's a quick introduction to one relaxation procedure. I call it, appropriately, the *quick release*. Read the directions first and then try it. Close your eyes, take a deep breath, and hold it as you tighten every muscle in your body that you can think of (your fists, arms, legs, stomach, neck, buttocks, etc.). Hold your breath, keeping your muscles tense, for about six seconds. Then let it out in a "whoosh," and allow the tension to drain out of your muscles. Let your body go limp. Keep your eyes closed, and breathe rhythmically and comfortably for about twenty seconds. Repeat this tension-relaxation cycle three times. By the end of the third repetition, you'll probably feel a lot more relaxed.

Pinpointing

Are you more comfortable now? Then you're ready to proceed to the next crucial step. In order to deal with anything that's upsetting you, you'll want to determine exactly what it is that's bothering you! Make a list. Then go over what you've written. In reviewing your list you'll see that just about every item can be placed into one of two categories. The first category contains the *modifiables*, or the things (whether problems or emotions) you *can* do something about. The second category includes the nonmodifiables, or things you *can't* do anything about. Why separate them? Because the two categories have different implications for dealing with them.

For the first category, you'll want to figure out what strategies you can use to improve the situation. You'll plan a course of action as soon as you identify exactly what's bothering you. How about the second category? You'll still be planning strategies, but of a different kind! Where do your emotions exist? In your mind, right? Therefore, your plan for this category is to work on the way you're thinking.

What Should You Do?

How can you change your thinking so that something will bother you less? The technique you use really depends on what emotional reaction is bothering you. For example, if you're afraid of something and you want to conquer this fear, a procedure called *systematic desensitization* may be helpful. We'll go into this later in the chapter on Fears and Anxieties.

If you're feeling guilty or angry about something, or if something is depressing you, it can be very helpful for you to learn how to change or "restructure" the way you're thinking. You'll learn more about techniques for that in the later chapters on Guilt, Anger, and Depression.

Actually, any of the procedures we've discussed can be used with just about any problem. It's just a question of deciding what's best for *you* in how you cope with your emotions.

WHAT ABOUT THE FUTURE?

Even if you do have intense emotional reactions, these will diminish, either because of the passage of time or because you're doing something to help. On the other hand, you'll experience more emotional reactions when your symptoms are more pronounced. So you'll probably experience a range of emotional reactions from time to time. But even when these feelings do occur, you can usually point to so many positive things going on in your life—so many ways that you can recognize progress—that it's not such a difficult thing to deal with.

Although emotions do not cause rheumatoid arthritis, they can certainly interfere with your ability to live with the disease. In addition, emotional upsets can, in some cases, exacerbate your condition. So doesn't it make sense to do what you can to control your emotions?

The purpose of this section is to help you to understand the different emotions you may experience. You'll discover where they come from and, very importantly, recognize that many others have gone through exactly what you're going through. In addition, a number of strategies will be presented to help you cope with these emotions more effectively. Remember that "practice makes perfect." Just reading about a method to control an emotion doesn't mean you'll experience instant success. You have to keep practicing.

In the following chapters you'll see how these different techniques can be used. So don't be afraid, depressed, guilty, or angry! Instead, read on!

7

Coping With The Diagnosis

When you first found out you had RA, how did you feel? How did you react when your doctor finally told you the news? Your initial reaction could probably fit neatly into one of two categories.

REACTION 1: PANIC ATTACK!

One type of reaction (certainly not a pleasant one) is terror. Sheer panic! "I'm too young for this!" "On no, what's going to happen to me?" "How will the disease affect me?" "Will I ever be 'normal?'" "What is the treatment (and how will I handle it)?" "Am I going to be confined to a wheelchair?" "Will I ever get better?" "Who will take care of me?" "Am I going to be crippled for life?" These are all tense questions that may pop up when you're diagnosed. Family members and loved ones may ask them (and panic) as well. You may think that your life may never be the same again. For life will now include treatment for RA.

Let's talk about this reaction. Does anyone you know like pain or physical restrictions? No way. It's normal to be afraid. You may suddenly be hit with the fact that you are mortal and vulnerable. You'll realize you may have this problem for the rest of your life. Physically, it's not uncommon to feel faint, a shortness of breath, or to experience other stress reactions at the time of diagnosis.

REACTION 2: WHAT A RELIEF!

The other type of reaction is that of relief. Now that may seem strange to you! Why would you be relieved to know that you have RA? Well, perhaps you were experiencing a lot of pain and nothing seemed to help. Maybe your family and friends didn't believe you, and thought the problem was all in your head! You might have thought you had a fatal illness (some people actually feel this way!), and were relieved to find out that you weren't dying. At least knowing what the cause is can be a relief.

If you *were* relieved after your diagnosis, you probably had a much easier time coping with the start of treatment. Why? One reason is because you're hopeful that treatment will significantly improve the way you've been feeling (and it's good to finally know *why* you're feeling that way). Second, family members and friends who may not have believed that you were really sick will now discover the truth. Unfortunately, some people close to you may still not believe that the problem is physical. They may continue to believe that the problem is either emotional or stress-related. You can't force everyone to believe a medical diagnosis! However, most doubts will probably disappear. Strained relationships may improve. Family members may sometimes feel guilty as they realize that they have been skeptical about your condition. They may have criticized your inability to fulfill responsibilities and your decreased ability to do things. They did this because they thought a real illness did not exist. Now they know the truth! Third, and most important, you'll be relieved that it wasn't all in your head. After a long period of time, even the most confident person can begin to wonder whether or not there was really something wrong or if it was purely emotional.

WHY MIGHT I FEEL CALM?

Frequently, as with any traumatic event, you may feel numb at first. You may sit quietly in the doctor's office, listening to everything that is being said. But you may not really be absorbing it. You may hear your doctor talking, but his words are not penetrating. You might even actively and calmly participate in the discussion, without any emotional reaction. That may come later!

HOW ABOUT DENIAL?

Denying that a problem exists is not unusual. Regardless of what symptoms you've been experiencing, hearing that you have RA may provoke denial. You may protest, "Oh, you're just making that up," "I don't have this problem the way you think I do," "Why don't you give it a little more time—I'm sure the problem will go away by itself," or even "#! (*) x#—leave me alone!"

If you're reading this book, then chances are you're probably not denying your condition. But if you *are* denying, the best way to start coping with your situation is to face reality. Speak to those professionals who know about your condition and have them explain it in further detail. Let them explain why treatment is necessary. Look at any x-rays that have been taken. Talk to other people with RA and listen to what they went through when they were first diagnosed. You will find that many of their experiences parallel your own. You may also discover self-help groups that can add to your knowledge of RA, as well as your coping ability.

Did you ever ask yourself, "Why can't I go back to the way things used to be?" Have you ever wished you could wake up one morning and find out that this was all a bad dream? The more you keep hoping that it will go away, the more you are slowing down your adjustment. Why is this so? Because you're not really admitting to yourself that you've changed—perhaps permanently. Rather, you're trying to push it out of your mind, hoping that things will return to the way they were. Such denial can obviously make it hard to cope with having RA, since the problem is not being faced realistically. Try to recognize that your condition does exist now, that it affects you, and that it will remain with you. Try to plan all your activities and aim all your thinking towards the notion that you are going to do what you can to handle it effectively.

DEATH WISH

Did you ever wish you could die after being told you have RA? Some people do. Emotionally, they exclaim that they'd rather die than have to go through this. If you've ever felt this way, don't feel guilty about such thoughts. You're not alone. Although you may feel like giving up from time to time, these feelings can go away if you work hard enough on them.

HOW DO YOU START TO ADJUST?

You must help yourself. Sure, you can receive love and support from your family and friends, and you can get expertise and support from professionals. But that's never enough. *You* are the one who is going to have to come to grips with your condition. This is something you have to do yourself, regardless of what anyone else says or does. At first, adjusting may be a very difficult and ongoing struggle. It may require a lot of effort and understanding. You may go through a lot of emotional turmoil, but there is no other way out. You must face it.

Information, please! Get as much of it as you can. Most of your initial reactions probably occurred because you didn't know enough about RA. So you'll want to learn as much as possible. Your physician will be helpful in providing information, or will at least suggest ways of getting it. Read a lot, but make sure that your reading material is current.

After reading general, consumer-oriented information, you might want to move on to more technical material. Ask questions about anything you don't understand. It probably wasn't a life-long goal of yours to become an expert on RA, but think about how much this can help you. Doctors will respect your questions more. And you'll understand exactly what's going on in your body. These are just two of the many advantages that can come from reading about your condition.

Support services and organizations such as the Arthritis Foundation have the specific purpose of providing you with current information on RA. Not only does the Arthritis Foundation have reading material, but it sponsors forums, symposia, speakers, arthritis clubs, and arthritis self-help classes all designed to help you.

Beware of Less Reputable Sources

Should you believe everything you read? Of course not. You may come across "cures" in weekly newspapers or magazines that sound incredible; alternatives for proper treatment that make you regret having started it in the first place. Or you may read in a glossy, weekly magazine that snake venom was successful in eliminating all RA symptoms! (Don't count on it!) Make sure that whatever you read is reputable, and remember that it takes rigorous scientific study before one can prove that a new procedure or treatment is actually effective. And be sensible. If some exciting new treatment or medication were discovered, wouldn't you expect to learn about it in your daily newspaper or on a national news program? More about this later, in the chapter on quackery.

Dealing With Your Emotional Reactions

Begin working consciously to control any anxiety or stress that's making you feel less than comfortable. Once you have accepted the fact that you have a chronic illness and you'll have to alter your lifestyle, you'll want to try to control as many harmful emotions as you can.

It's very easy for your imagination to run wild. You'll probably keep thinking about all the things that can possibly go wrong. You'll worry about every symptom. So learn the facts about your condition.

This is a great way to alleviate some of the anxiety caused by the diagnosis.

The emotions stemming from any chronic condition can be unpleasant. You may engage in prolonged periods of regret, sorrow, and nostalgia, remembering the way it used to be. Many fears come to mind, some of which can be overwhelming. Fear of incapacitation, of being handicapped, of losing friends—all are very understandable fears. Begin facing them. They can and must be faced in order to move your adjustment along more smoothly. Speak to other people who have RA. Learn how they've adjusted. This can be very helpful.

WHAT'S NEXT?

Once you've become more familiar with your condition, and understand how if affects you, what can you do to deal with it? For one thing, learn what specific changes may have to be made in your lifestyle. There is no way of knowing how many changes you'll have to make, but you do want to create the best possible life for yourself.

Obviously, work with a physician you can trust—one who has had experience working with people with RA before. It's usually recommended that people with RA be treated by a board-certified rheumatologist. But you still want to find a physician you feel comfortable with. Remember that the patient-physician relationship you develop now will be helpful in your life with RA later on.

How About the Family?

A very important part of adjusting to the diagnosis of RA is for your family to learn to adjust as well. It's hard for everyone if those around you have difficulty accepting your condition. But dealing with the diagnosis can be hard for family members. They, too, will go through periods of denial when they will say, "No, everything will be fine" or "I'm sure the problem will clear up by itself."

Ann Marie, a 34-year-old nurse, had only recently been diagnosed as having RA. After a few depressing weeks, however, she began to learn how to cope. She was finally able to handle thoughts of lifestyle changes, concerns about reduced mobility, and some of the other unpleasant thoughts associated with RA. Sound great? Not really. You see, her husband of fourteen years couldn't admit she had a problem, her children were afraid she was going to die, and even her 68-year-old mother was considering selling her ranch in Texas to move closer. Although Ann Marie was learning how to cope with RA, she could not cope with her family. They couldn't handle it, and were making things very difficult for her.

It's a great idea for family members to seek out people to speak to. They, too, can find out more about RA and about how others cope with treatment. Family members can follow the same suggestions given before: seeking self-help groups, speaking to physicians, and reading. So encourage family members and any willing friends to learn as much as they can. This will help your adjustment.

IN A NUTSHELL

Start thinking positively about your life with RA. Learn as much as you can about your condition. Use whatever support systems are necessary to help you. Use all the stress management and emotional control procedures available. Start saying to yourself, ''RA may be affecting me, but I'm still alive and I'm going to do whatever I can to help myself adjust to this.'' If it's necessary for you to make changes in your lifestyle—even major ones—tell yourself that you will make them, and you will make them willingly! You are going to lead as complete a life as you can. The more quickly you can adjust your lifestyle to fit your needs, the more rapidly you will be able to enjoy your life. This may be hard at first and will take time. But at least be grateful that you're not helpless, and can take steps to make the most of your life with RA!

8

Depression

Bill was depressed. A 49-year-old father of three, he had been married for twenty-four years and lived in a beautiful ranch house in a well-to-do neighborhood. It looked as though he had everything he could ever ask for—except a life without RA! And oh, what an effect this had on him! In the past, Bill had always been enthusiastic about life. But he now became extremely unhappy whenever he thought about the future. He felt that he could never participate in sports again, and was afraid he would end up confined to a wheelchair. He didn't even want to spend time with his children. Yes, Bill was suffering from depression.

Depression is a serious problem. The very mention of the word can sometimes knock the smile right off your face. Actual numbers vary, but it is estimated that more than two million Americans need professional care for depression. Because it is so widespread, depression has been nicknamed the "common cold" of emotional problems.

Just what is depression? Depression is an extremely unpleasant feeling of unhappiness and despair. It can range from mild (where you may feel discouraged and downhearted) to severe (where you can feel utterly hopeless, worthless, and unwilling to go on living). You may feel that there is no reason to remain a part of the world.

Depression can be painful. Imagine how it must hurt to feel (or say), "I wish I were never born. What good am I? I'm not helping anybody around me and I'm not helping myself." It may seem like life and the world are against you. Life is unfair. It is a constant struggle in which you never win. That hurts.

DEPRESSION AFFECTS YOUR BODY

The more noticeable symptoms of depression may be physical. Nervous activity or agitation, such as wringing of the hands, may occur. You may be restless, or have difficulty remaining in one place. On the other hand, you may become much less active, and remain motionless for abnormally long periods of time (appearing almost in a trance, with no apparent desire to do anything). Bill's wife, Marie, became very concerned when her husband remained sitting in a chair in the living room for hours at a time. When she asked him a question he would respond in monosyllables. When friends called on the phone, he never wanted to talk to them. Bill's depression was causing him to lose interest in just about everything.

Other physical changes that can occur are a reduction or increase in appetite, a decreased interest in sex, and, for some women, cessation of menstruation. If you're mildly depressed, you may have difficulty concentrating, and your attention span may be much shorter. Guys may remain unshaven simply because they don't feel like shaving. When you speak (and you'll probably do less of that, too) your conversation will usually be shallow, emphasizing feelings of worthlessness and despair. Most of your physical activities will also slow down (and not just because of RA restrictions).

You'll probably feel exhausted. This may seem surprising, since you're not doing much of anything anyway. But constantly telling yourself that you're no good can be very tiring! You really don't want to believe this, but you feel like you have no choice. In attempting to escape these feelings you may become even more depressed, as well as more physically drained and exhausted.

Depression may cause you to feel physically sick. This is because of the many ways your body reacts when you're depressed. Any of the symptoms we've talked about thus far might be related to a physical disorder. But if the symptoms go away when your depression improves, don't just assume that they're related to the depression. A medical examination may still be a good idea. This way, you'll be sure that there is no organic disease causing your depression.

DEPRESSION AFFECTS YOUR MOOD

You may experience frequent mood swings. For example, you might feel worse in the morning and better in the evening. This may be because of joint stiffness and pain, as well as depression. Another reason why you may feel better in the evening is because you realize that it's almost time to go to sleep—a means of escape. But depression may also cause difficulty sleeping, even if you weren't doing much of anything during the day.

When you're depressed, you feel like your mood keeps getting "lower." You like yourself very little, if at all. Your thinking is very negative—very different from the way it is when you're feeling good.

It is your negative thinking (not just a particular triggering event) that leads to your depression. This negative thinking tends to be the most frequently overlooked and misunderstood part of depression. Recognizing this is an important first step in learning to cope with depression.

DEPRESSION AFFECTS RELATIONSHIPS WITH OTHERS

If you're depressed, you may feel that people around you have no need for you. As Bill used to complain, "Why should my friends want to see me or make plans with me? I can't do anything!"

Do you feel less at ease talking to others? Does it seem like others are having a hard time talking to you, even if they have been close to you for a long time? Because of your depression, you may be less interested in conversation, and less confident. You may project *your* feelings of self-worthlessness onto others, believing that they really don't want to talk to you. The more depressed you are, the more persuasive you may be in convincing other people around you that you are no good.

Ann received a telephone call from her friend Susan. Susan wanted to know how Ann had been feeling, since the last time they had gotten together Ann seemed to be in a great deal of pain. Ann responded half-heartedly, sensing that Susan was only calling out of obligation. She then explained that she would understand if Susan did not want to call again, since she never seemed to have any good news to tell her. How do you think Susan felt? Imagine hearing this repeatedly, despite reassuring Ann that her concern was sincere. Would you be surprised if, eventually, Susan got tired of even trying, and probably stopped calling? But in Ann's mind, this would only reinforce the fact that she really was no good, and that she was not worthy of having any friends after all!

DEPRESSION AFFECTS PHYSICAL ACTIVITIES

Do you find that you are getting less satisfaction from your normal activities? Are you functioning like a robot? Does it seem like something is missing? It can be depressing to realize that something you used to enjoy no longer gives you the same pleasure, especially if you don't know why. It almost seems like there is a force propelling you to "go through the motions," while your heart just isn't in it. It is understandable, therefore, that if you are depressed, you might prefer to withdraw from such activities. What happens after that first depressing event occurs? A kind of chain reaction follows. This one occurrence creates a feeling that spreads like wildfire. It's almost as if the bottom has dropped out of your world. You may feel less able to control your thinking (although this is not true, as we will see later). But keep in mind: the deeper you go into depression, the harder it is to climb back out again. Therefore, you certainly want to catch these feelings of depression as early as possible, to try and keep yourself from spiraling further downward.

WHAT CAUSES DEPRESSION?

Where does depression come from? Sometimes we can figure this out, and sometimes we can't. But before we give up, let's discuss some of the possible causes.

How About the Normal "Downs?"

A certain amount of depression is normal in anyone's life. Nobody's life is a constant "upper." We all experience normal cycles of ups and downs. If we never experienced some of the downs, how could we ever fully appreciate the ups!? However, when depression becomes more than just the "normal downs," then it must be attended to. Nipping it quickly in the bud can keep it from becoming much worse.

There are certain things in anyone's life that can understandably lead to depression. Certain traumatic experiences such as losing a loved one, being diagnosed with a chronic illness, requiring major surgery, being fired from a job—all may certainly lead to depression. That would be understandable. However, this *doesn't* mean you should ignore the problem or wait until it goes away. It's essential to learn how to deal with depression, since this is so important in learning how to cope with RA.

How About Anger You Can't Express?

What if you get so angry that you feel like you're going to burst? But you don't (or can't) do anything about it, so you decide to "swallow" it. It seems strange that a powerful feeling like anger can turn into a withdrawn, helpless feeling like depression. But it's true. If you become increasingly angry about something and feel unable to do anything about it, you may turn the anger inward. You may feel so much frustration or hopelessness that you "shut down" in an attempt to keep yourself from these terrible feelings. This leads to withdrawal, which is a symptom of depression.

Is It All In Our Minds?

A small percentage of depression cases may be caused by biochemical deficiencies—some chemical imbalance in our bodies. This does not occur very often, however. Treatment for biochemical deficiencies may involve the administration of drugs in an effort to re-balance the chemicals in our bodies. This usually isn't the whole answer. But regardless of whether your depression is caused by this or, more typically, by your reactions to things, people, and events around you, you should still try to modify your behavior and improve your thinking. Many experts believe that even if the cause of depression *is* biochemical, by working on improving your thoughts and behaviors you *can* have a positive effect on your depression.

How About Rheumatoid Arthritis?

Can RA cause depression? Are you kidding??? Living with RA can certainly create depression or magnify already-existing depression.

The depression you felt after being diagnosed with RA is understandable. But it can get better as you begin to adjust to your new life situation. There's a problem, though. Because life with RA has its ups and downs (physically), your feelings may bounce up and down as well. This can be a problem, considering what depression can do to you.

You may be saying to yourself, "If I'm depressed over my RA, how can I expect to get over my depression unless I get rid of this disease?" That kind of thinking will get you nowhere. Even if you go into remission, you still can't ignore the fact that your RA is a chronic condition. So if your depression lingers, don't wait. Work on it. Learn how to cope with it. We'll talk more later about how you can improve your thinking.

What else about RA might depress you? You might become depressed thinking about the future, not knowing what your prognosis is or how it will affect your life. Knowing that you need supportive devices can be depressing, as well as the fact that you'll probably need medication to keep your condition from getting worse. Changes in habits necessitated by your condition and its treatment may also be depressing.

Problems involving other people may depress you. You may feel helpless at not being able to share what you're experiencing or the way you feel. You may get depressed if others don't understand what you're going through. You may be depressed over the possibility of damaged relationships, lost friendships, or family friction. If you're single, you may become depressed thinking that you'll never meet anyone or be able to develop a meaningful relationship because of the changes in your life necessitated by RA.

WHAT MAINTAINS DEPRESSION?

You may be blaming yourself (or your RA) for everything that is wrong. You may tend to become more and more withdrawn, and pull away from the world around you. Why? Well, if you believe that your condition is causing all these horrible things, isn't it better to "escape" and not think about it? Realistically, escaping doesn't solve anything. But if you're depressed, you may feel that withdrawal is the only way to solve this dilemma. This keeps you depressed (in fact, it can make you even more depressed).

Although you may seem sullen and withdrawn to others, you're probably in deep emotional pain. Part of what makes you, and keeps you, depressed is your failure to protect yourself from this emotional pain. When your mind does allow any thoughts to enter, you tend to feel overwhelmed by feelings of doom and destruction. You feel that nothing good can possibly happen—that only bad things can happen. So what do you do? You try to block everything out of your mind!

So why do you stay depressed? Why doesn't it just go away? It may be because you don't want to talk to anybody, or to even consider therapy. Therefore, the thoughts and feelings leading to your depression tend to be kept hidden. You may ask, "Is my unwillingness to talk the only reason why I'm still depressed? If I start talking more, will that get me out of my depression?" Not necessarily. But it can be helpful to talk out your feelings. It would probably be helpful (even though you wouldn't be too thrilled) if a close friend or family member took the initiative and forced you into some kind of conversation (therapeutic or otherwise) or, at least, into doing something physical.

HOW DO WE DEAL WITH DEPRESSION?

Can anything be done? Of course! Would I abandon you without any suggestions? First, tell yourself that the *main* reason why you're still depressed is because you have not yet taken the proper steps toward feeling better! These steps can "bring you out of the rut" and reacquaint you with the more positive, pleasant aspects of living that you'd like to experience. Don't think it's easy, though. Unfortunately, once you've fallen into depression, it takes effort, hard work, and a certain amount of persistence to pull yourself back up. The fight however, is surely worth it. Of course, the fight can be made easier if you know of specific techniques and activities that will help.

Once you feel better, you're not going to ever want to feel that depressed again, right? Well, the strategies and techniques that are most effective in dealing with depression can also be effective in preventing you from becoming depressed again! This doesn't mean you'll *never* feel depressed again. It may happen. Anticipate it, so that if it does recur, you won't completely fall apart. And if it does happen, won't it be good to know that you can fight it? You *can* do something to help yourself!

Depression Treatment

Now that you're ready to fight your depression, consider two major ways of dealing with it: being more physical (in other words, *doing* something), and working on your thinking.

It can be very helpful to make a list of all the things that are depressing you. You may feel there'll be at least fifty items! But in actuality, you'll probably start running dry after six or seven. Then divide this list into two more lists: first, things that you *can* do something about, and second, things you *can't* do anything about. Sound familiar? You read about this earlier in the section. But it really works for a number of different problems. Get physical (do something) about those items in the first list, and get thoughtful (work on your thinking) regarding those items in the second list.

Let's Get Physical

Unknowingly, you may be using a lot of energy to keep yourself depressed. You may be working hard to keep that anger inside, even if it appears to others that you are withdrawing. If your depression is anger turned within, then we can logically assume that, by releasing it, feelings of depression can be eliminated. But what do you do with those feelings? You must find an object towards which your anger can be expressed. This may be difficult. However, it's important to release the trapped anger so that it doesn't build up further and deepen the depression.

Have you ever been in this situation? You're sitting there, depressed and withdrawn. Somebody makes an innocent remark, and you practically snap the person's head off! What's happening? Whatever was said triggered the release of the internalized anger that was making you depressed. Look out, world!

Consider for a moment all the energy that is keeping you depressed. You've read about why it is important to release this energy outwardly. What kinds of activities can be helpful for this? Many types of intense physical activity can release this energy. But although getting physical may improve your depression, it's your thoughts that make you depressed. Physical activity can provide a great distraction, which can help you to look more objectively at what's going on. That will help. But it may not teach you what you need the most: ways of fighting inappropriate thinking. Besides, RA may not even allow you to participate in intense physical activity! Fortunately, this isn't the only way to lift depression.

Let's Get Thoughtful

So if you can "think" yourself into depression, you can obviously "think" yourself out of it. How? Your thoughts show how you "talk to yourself." In fact, when it comes to talking to yourself, you're probably the biggest chatterbox you know! But if you're depressed, you're just talking yourself down. All your comments (or at least most of them) are probably put-downs; harsh statements offering little to be happy about. These can make you feel even worse. You want your inner voice to help you, not hurt you. Let's see how you can do that.

Distinguishing Fact From Fiction

Don't get defensive when I tell you this: when you're depressed, you tend to distort reality. Clinical research with depressed patients has proven this. Recognize, therefore, that your thoughts are not necessarily based on what is really going on, but on your own distorted views. This is called *cognitive distortion*.

Is that bad? You bet your happiness it is. "Cognitive" refers to your thinking. "Distortion" means you're twisting things around and, in general, losing sight of what's real. We all tend to do this from time to time. But when you're depressed, you do it a *lot*, if not *all* the time, and it *keeps* you depressed. So how do you stop? First, you must become reacquainted with what is really happening, and with the facts. But how can you do that if you keep distorting reality? Right now, you're better off accepting somebody *else's* perceptions of the situation, because that person is probably a lot more objective and accurate. Since so many feelings of worthlessness are based on distorted facts, depression can be reduced, if not eliminated, once these facts are straightened out.

Monique kept moaning because none of her friends were calling her. "They don't call as much as they used to. I guess they just don't care." Her sister, Andrea, asked her to estimate how often her friends used to call. When Monique compared this number to the current number of calls she was receiving, she realized that the numbers were almost the same. She then realized that she was probably just more sensitive because of all the changes going on in her life! Although she did not feel 100% better, it was good to know that she wasn't being abandoned.

Making Molehills Out Of Mountains

Does this imply that if you're depressed you have no real problems? Is it "all in your head?" No. Everyone has problems. If you feel good, you can handle them, but if you're depressed, you may feel overwhelmed. Each and every part of your life, regardless of how trivial or slight it may be, tends to depress you. As the depression lifts, you will again be able to deal with all of life's problems—big and small.

Self-Fulfilling Prophecy

We've discussed several different ways that you may feel if you're depressed. Are all these feelings irrational and untrue? No. Ironically, although some of them may start off being far from the truth, the longer you feel that way the more chance there will be for them to become "self-fulfilling prophecies." In other words, you'll begin convincing yourself that nonsense makes sense. For example, if you begin telling yourself that friends and relatives don't care, this may become a reality because your negative attitudes may alienate the people close to you. They may decide it's not worth the bother. As far as your activities go, you are less likely to do anything when you're depressed. You'll probably be less likely to even attempt doing things that you used to enjoy. As a result, you'll feel less competent and will not accomplish anything. This just tends to magnify and confirm your feelings of worthlessness, leading to even greater depression. Not a pretty picture.

Once you begin feeling depressed, your negative thoughts will soon lead to negative actions. These negative actions will lead to more negative thoughts, which will in turn lead to more negative actions, and so on. It is an ongoing, vicious cycle that will spiral you further downward into deeper depression. Eventually you'll feel trapped in this vicious cycle, with no way to escape from the "dumps."

Are you getting depressed just reading this? In all probability, if you've ever been depressed, you've said to yourself at least once already, "Wow, that sounds just like me!" So you see, your negative thoughts become self-fulfilling prophecies. If you find that you are starting to believe in your negative thoughts, stop yourself. Try to think positive thoughts, so that if your thought *does* turn out to be real, it will at least be a positive one.

Positive is the Opposite of Negative

As we've said before, depression results from—and causes—a lot of negative thinking. Negative thoughts automatically pop into your mind and you cannot stop them. It's like trying to keep your eyes open when you sneeze! You just can't do it. But once you become aware of them, then you *can* do something. People who remain depressed feel incapable of doing anything about their negative thinking and allow these thoughts to continue. They simply continue in that vicious, downward cycle that was mentioned earlier.

Alice, a 34-year-old housewife, was resting when the telephone rang. "I'm sure that's Katherine, calling to cancel our lunch plans," she thought to herself. Within the thirty seconds it took her to get to the phone, she had become so depressed that she considered not even answering the call. Imagine how she felt when she reluctantly answered the phone and discovered that it was a wrong number! Alice had allowed her negative thoughts to run wild—she became more and more negative until she was about ready to give up. And for what? There was no clear-cut reason for thinking the way she did.

Once she realized that she was thinking this way, what should she have done? She should have *countered* her thoughts. She should have told herself, "It may not even be Katherine on the phone. Or if it is, maybe she's just calling to confirm. I won't let it bother me now. After all, I don't even know who it is!" This is the beginning of positive thinking.

Dwell on the Brighter Tomorrows

If you find yourself unhappily comparing your present life to life before RA, try to modify your thinking. Start planning fun things for the present and future. Anyone can come up with some enjoyable things to do, regardless of how restricted you may be. But it takes effort. Don't wallow in self-pity, because that will allow your depression to strangle you. Work on your thinking, develop some positive plans, and translate them into pleasure. Then wave goodbye to your depression!

When you recall the past, you may not even think it was that much better. You may have had other physical problems. You may have made some mistakes in your life. This may make you even more depressed about the future. However, you can't change the past. What's done is done. Keep telling yourself that. Tell yourself that you're going to work on making the future better. Set up some specific goals, starting with the easy-to-reach ones. You'll be helping yourself just by thinking about what you can do that's more positive. Don't punish yourself for the past.

What's Missing From Your Life?

You may have laughed when you read the title of this section. "Good health," you might respond. "Mobility without pain!" Sure. But why discuss this? Because depressed people frequently lament the fact that something is missing from their lives. What is usually missing is a feeling of satisfaction, accomplishment, and pride that normally comes from others' praise. You may just miss the attention and interest of other people. This may cause you to feel worthless. How do you counteract this? Think about your positive qualities (yes, you do have some!). Think about how you can interact more with people, spark their interest, and obtain more of the satisfaction that makes you feel worthwhile.

Shoot For the Earth, Not the Moon

We all have goals for ourselves. It's normal to become depressed when we don't reach a particular goal, especially if we've tried very hard to get there. But maybe it's not a realistic goal. Maybe you're trying to do something you can't, and you're getting depressed instead of realistically resetting your goal.

Arthur had not returned to work since a major flare had knocked him flat on his back several weeks ago. Finally, after a long period of rest and medication, he was feeling better and was looking forward to getting back to work so he could catch up on everything. When his doctor finally gave him the "go ahead," he practically flew to his office. After two hours of phone calls, consultations, dictation, and meetings, he was exhausted. His feelings plummeted. He became worried that he wouldn't be able to handle all the pressure, and that he was in danger of losing his job. Wrong! Arthur had simply set his sights too high. Expecting to return to his old schedule as if he didn't have RA was just not realistic. Try to return to your old activities slowly. Build up your stamina. Isn't the end result more important? And if your goals are more realistically set, you'll have a much better chance of achieving them, and less of a chance of falling short.

AN ANTI-DEPRESSING SUMMARY

The best way to work on negative thoughts is to prevent them from continuing. Be more realistically positive. Deal with reality the way it actually exists. Deal with thoughts from a more factual point of view. Deal with them the way somebody else might—somebody who is not depressed and who can be more objective. Try to make your perceptions more accurate, your awareness more realistic, and your thoughts more positive and constructive. Remember: Your thoughts lead to your emotions. If your thoughts are negative and critical, then your emotions will also be in bad shape. If you can turn your thoughts around to a more positive, constructive point of view, you'll see that your emotional reactions will improve as well.

9

Fears and Anxieties

Don't be "afraid" to read this chapter! It may help you discover what you're "anxious" about!

The two sentences above may help you to distinguish between fear and anxiety. What's the difference? *Anxiety* is a general sense of uneasiness; a vague feeling of discomfort. It is an agitated, uncertain state in which you just don't feel at peace or in control. There is a premonition that something bad may happen, which you have to protect yourself against. You feel very vulnerable. However, you're not exactly sure what the source of your anxiety is.

Fear, on the other hand, is usually more specific. It's often directed toward something that can be recognized, whether it's a person, object, situation, or event. We have fear when we become aware of something dangerous, or when we feel threatened. When we are afraid (as with feeling anxious) we also feel out of control and less confident. So the *feelings* of fear and anxiety are basically the same. The main difference is whether you can identify the source of the feeling. From this point on, however, I'll be using the two terms interchangeably so there is less confusion.

Fear is so prevalent that many words are used to describe it: scared, concerned, alarmed, worried, uptight, nervous, edgy, shaky. Then there's perplexed, wary, having cold feet, frightened, helpless, frustrated. Is that it? Nope! How about suspicious, keyed-up, impatient, giddy, hesitant, apprehensive, tense, panicky, disturbed, agitated? Of course, there are more, but if I went on this book would have to be renamed, "The Fear Synonym Book." All these words mean the same thing: "I'm afraid." The source of this fear may be real or imaginary.

IS FEAR GOOD OR BAD?

Believe it or not, fear is usually good! Now you're probably saying, "If I'm shaking with fear, how can it be good?" Fear mobilizes you. It "tells" you to prepare to attack the source of your fear. You react in a way that leads to action. In this regard, fear is similar to stress. It serves a necessary and critical purpose. In a way, it "protects" you.

Fear is bad only if it is denied, or if it is so excessive that you can't do anything about it. If you face it and push past it, trying to resolve it, then fear is a positive emotion. It is only when the source of fear becomes overlooked, ignored, or denied that the consequences may be a problem. This is because the threat or danger is allowed to continue, and nothing (or not enough) is being done to control it.

HOW INTENSE ARE OUR REACTIONS?

Fear ranges in intensity from mild to severe. It is impossible to measure how much fear there is in anyone's life. It is unique and varies from person to person.

What determines how fearful you get? Usually the strength of the feared object, person, or event is important. Also, how close is it (wouldn't you be more afraid of getting an injection within the next thirty seconds, than if you were getting it in thirty days)? How vulnerable are you (do you *hate* injections, or are you just tired of feeling like a pincushion)? How successful are you in defending yourself (can you calmly accept the needle, or do you scream a lot)? These are some of the factors determining how you handle fear. Your own strength and the success of your defense mechanisms also play a role.

People with rheumatoid arthritis can be afraid of many things. Obviously, the more fears you have, the more these can interfere with your successful adjustment. Recognizing your fears and learning how to deal with them will help you live more happily and more comfortably. How? I was afraid you'd never ask!

HOW TO COPE WITH FEARS AND ANXIETIES

The first step in coping with your fears is to use the "pinpointing" technique discussed earlier. List all the things you're afraid of. Identify exactly what you are afraid of and exactly why you are afraid. Then think about what you can do to alleviate your fears.

For Joyce, this was not hard. She knew she was afraid of how people would react when they saw she needed a cane to walk. She quickly realized that what she feared was rejection. She was concerned that they wouldn't want to be with her because of their own fears ("Could this happen to me?"). She planned a course of action (no, not a one-way ticket to Brazil!). She decided she'd simply do the best she could, expecting her friends to accept her the way she was. If they didn't, that was *their* loss. She was less afraid almost instantly. As you begin planning your strategies, and gradually put your plan into operation, you'll continue to feel better and better.

Desensitize Yourself

A great technique used to conquer fear is called *systematic desensitization*. You learn to desensitize yourself, to make yourself less vulnerable to the source of your fear.

Here's how you can try it. Sit in a comfortable chair and relax. Then create a movie in your mind. Imagine what it is that makes you afraid. If you get tense, stop imagining it and relax. When you've calmed down, try imagining it again. The more you try to imagine your fear, the less it will bother you. Try it! It will give you a great feeling of relaxation and control. There are several library books that provide more information on systematic desensitization. Check them out.

It was stated earlier that anxiety is a vague, uneasy feeling with an unknown source. So how can you cope with it by following the steps listed above? Well, if you try to pinpoint the source and are unable to, then you probably can't follow the steps. So what do you do? Use relaxation procedures. Work on changing your thinking. Even if you can't pinpoint a specific fear, these techniques will greatly help you to cope with general anxiety.

LET'S TALK ABOUT SPECIFICS

Remember, it is understandable for you to have many fears related to your condition. A problem arises, however, when you don't admit these fears. As a result, you don't do anything about resolving them. They *can* be resolved. And you *can* work on changing your thinking.

Initial Fears

When you were first diagnosed, many fearful questions probably came to mind. "What will the future be like? What will become of me? Will I need a wheelchair? Will I be crippled?" These are all legitimate questions and justifiable fears. But time goes on. Some of these questions have been answered, and some of your initial qualms have not materialized. But you're probably still afraid of some things. Let's discuss some of them.

Fear of Pain

Nobody likes pain. Pain is one of the most unpleasant problems associated with RA. You may be afraid of pain. This fear may be just as strong when you *don't* have pain, since you're afraid of it happening! If you do feel pain, you'll wonder when you're going to feel some relief. Each little twinge of pain may make you afraid of further deterioration of your condition, or that additional problems exist or may develop. What can you do about this fear? Try to accept the fact that some pain may be "with you" from time to time, but medication can reduce its intensity. Further suggestions will be offered in the chapter on Pain. Realize that each pain "cycle" will eventually stop or at least ease up. It *won't* last forever.

Fear of Medication and Possible Side Effects

You may be nervous about the different medication that you have to take, even though you need it. You may be afraid of what it's doing to your body. Just keep reminding yourself of what could happen without medication! Your physician is aware of the possible side effects, but will still prescribe medication, as long as the advantages of the medication outweigh the side effects.

Fear of "What Next?"

What will happen next? You can't be sure. Will there be an increase in the amount of pain? Will new joints become affected? Will you develop new side effects from your medication? Will you go into (or stay in) remission? When will your RA flare up? Fear of "what next?" includes being afraid of new symptoms, or the return of old ones.

Children may have lots of "what's next" fears. They may worry about completing school, getting a job, meeting friends, starting a family, and all the other things that children fear. But now JRA has compounded the problem. Children need to take life one day at a time (sound familiar?). If there's something that can be done (such as taking courses toward an appropriate job or career), that's the proper way to proceed. Otherwise, make the best out of what is.

Everyone *wonders* what's in store for the future. But because of the unpleasantness of what you've experienced, you may be *afraid* of the future, rather than merely curious. What can you do? Unless you own a crystal ball, you can't foresee what will happen in the future. So take life one day at a time. What will be, will be. (What a great name for a song!) Just tell yourself that you'll handle any problems as they occur.

Fear of Disability

The thought of being disabled may be horrible. Because RA can be physically restricting, you may have this fear. But being "disabled" is a bad term, since it suggests that you can't do *anything*. If you look around you or think more objectively, you'll realize that a physical disability wouldn't make you any less of a human being. You would still have many, many capabilities. Numerous Olympic champions began their athletic careers to overcome physical disabilities. Beethoven wrote some of his greatest music after becoming totally deaf. There was even a one-armed baseball player in the major leagues. Regardless of their disabilities, these people have one thing in common: the knowledge that they can overcome or at least compensate for a limitation in one area by developing abilities in another.

How might a disability affect you? One example is a tendency to become increasingly dependent on others, since you can't do as much for yourself. Once again, it's your thinking that's making you afraid. Other than trying to take good care of yourself, what else can you really do? Take things as they come, but think more positively. Remember: You still have lots of room for self-fulfillment.

If you are already disabled, this can certainly be frightening, especially if you enjoy independence. You don't want to be a burden to those important people in your life. Can you do anything about this? That depends on the nature of your disability. Find out everything you can about the possibility of rehabilitation. If there's any chance, take advantage of it. Even if there's no possibility of total rehabilitation, every little bit helps. Just don't let yourself collapse, or you'll be doing yourself an enormous disservice.

Fear of Being Crippled or In A Wheelchair

Fear of being crippled crosses the mind of most people with RA at one time or another. But be assured that a great majority of the people with RA will *not* become crippled, although your activities may be limited from time to time.

Just as unlikely are the chances of your ending up in a wheelchair. This would happen only if your joints were very severely damaged (usually because of neglect in careful treatment programs, or being in a location where adequate treatment is not available). Advances in modern medicine continue to decrease the chances of being crippled or ending up in a wheelchair. (This doesn't mean that, on a trip to Walt Disney World or the like, you wouldn't welcome a wheelchair as a support device!)

Fear of Falling

A very common fear for people with RA is that of falling down. There are two main reasons for this fear. First, you certainly don't want to hurt yourself. You may be afraid that, if you fall, you'd really do a lot of damage. And second, you may be afraid that, once you fall, you wouldn't be able to get back up!

What can you do? Try to be as careful as possible. Try to avoid hasty movements. Reorganize your living environment to reduce the chances of tripping over anything. Beyond this, however, remind yourself that you can only do so much. You don't want to fall. But if it happens, it happens, and you'll deal with it then!

Fear of Others' Reactions

Are you afraid that other people will not accept you with rheumatoid arthritis? Do you fear being shunned? You may fear rejection if you can't socialize the way you'd like to be able to. Others may feel you can't keep up with them. But don't try, because pushing yourself can be a painful way to maintain a friendship.

Unfortunately, some people can be cold and unfeeling and may have trouble dealing with you the way you are. Who needs those kinds of friends anyway? Other friends will accept you under any circumstances. Enjoy them. But since you can't change the way some people feel, try not to be as concerned with their reactions. Instead, be more attentive to your own needs and feelings.

Other fears in this category can be even more frightening. "What if my spouse leaves me? What if all my friends stay away from me?" Isolation can be a horrible thought. If it's not happening now, you may be afraid of it happening in the future. You may be afraid that none of your friends will remain "in your corner." To reduce the chances of such rejection, you may hesitate to make plans with friends or family. This would only add to your feeling of isolation.

Consider your thoughts, but be realistic. Remember that a change in a social relationship can occur for *any* reason, not just because of your condition! If you feel that your relationship is in jeopardy, see what you can do to help ("put all your cards on the table," discuss problems, even get counseling, if need be). But you can only do so much. If that doesn't work, even though the outcome may upset you, at least you know you've tried.

Fear of Overdoing/Underdoing

You may not know how much you should do. You may be afraid of doing too much, but you may feel guilty about doing too little! How do you conquer this? Get advice from experts. You need professional advice in coming up with the best "mix" of rest and exercise. This may become apparent only through trial-and-error. You can only learn through experience. Pace yourself. Change your level of activity gradually. Then tell yourself, as with so many other fears, that you're doing the best you can.

Fear of Employment Problems

You may be concerned about whether or not you'll be able to keep your job. You may want to work, but fear that you won't be able to. Your employer may be understanding at first, but you worry about how long this will continue. And, of course, you may be afraid of all the money problems that might result if you can't work. Can you do much to change the nature of fear? You can evaluate your vocational skills and make sure you have a job that you can handle. Other than this, you'll have to live with this fear, and just hope for the best. If there's a problem, you'll cope. Being afraid won't help.

Fear of Traveling

You may be reluctant to travel with RA. Why? You wouldn't know the doctors, what medical facilities were available, or whom you could contact if you experienced a problem. Obviously, if you travel by car, this may not be as much of a problem. But you may not be sure you can walk as much as you'd like, or if your destinations are conducive to your getting around.

What can you do? By planning in advance, you should be able to conquer this fear. Ask your doctor if he knows of any doctors or facilities where you're planning to go. You might want to contact them in advance. If your physician has no contacts, try to get some names either on your own (try the local medical society, or your local chapter of the Arthritis Foundation), or plan your vacation at a place where adequate medical services are available. Plan on not overdoing. Visiting five landmarks in one day is a bit much! (More about this in the chapter on travel.)

Fear of Loss of Income

Because of all your financial obligations, you need money! If you can't work, this pressure is even greater. Medical bills have to be paid. You can't depend on insurance plans, since they don't always provide enough coverage. In addition, many insurance plans require you to pay the doctor first and then get reimbursed. Doctors' fees can be quite high, and if the money is not coming in. . . . What can you do? Talk to people. Speak to others with RA who cannot work. See what they do. Maybe you'll get some ideas that will help you to conquer this fear.

Fear of Treatment Troubles

What if you've had problems with your treatment? It seems like you experience unpleasant side effects with every medication you've tried. Any therapy you've tried hasn't seemed to have done any good. You begin to fear that "nothing's gonna work." Yes, there are some people who have more difficulty than others finding the right "formula." And it's possible you may not benefit as much as you (or your doctor, family, therapists, friends, etc.) would like. But hang in there. New medication and techniques are being developed all the time. And, who knows? More trial-and-error may just come up with a solution. Giving up just makes you more tense and uncomfortable, anyway. So keep trying.

Fear of Dying

Because having a chronic illness means you are vulnerable, this fear is not uncommon. When might you be most afraid of dying? Probably at the time of diagnosis. That's when you feel the most vulnerable. Beginning a new treatment, or being involved in any of the ups and downs that remind you of your vulnerability, can also cause these fears. When you *feel* the worst, you're more likely to *fear* the worst. However, being afraid of dying is not going to help you feel better or live longer. If anything, it's only going to make you feel worse! Being afraid of dying, therefore, falls into the category of fears that you can do little or nothing about. How do you attack this fear? Research is constantly exploring new and improved treatment possibilities for individuals with RA. Improved surgical techniques, better technology, and new medical knowledge have significantly reduced the chances of serious consequences. So think positively. Others have had worse symptoms and still live comfortably. Do you see how you must work on your thinking? If negative thoughts make you *more* afraid, then positive thoughts . . . !

Fear of Not Coping

You may feel that you're barely handling having RA. You may think that any new problem that comes along will be enough to push you over the edge. Fear of falling apart can easily lead to panic; an out-of-control kind of feeling that *will* make you fall apart. Get a hold of yourself. Pinpoint those particular things you're having difficulty with, and get help in dealing with them. Don't wait. Don't project a false sense of bravado that you can and must handle everything yourself. If you feel yourself near the edge, get someone to help you to steady yourself. Talk it over with someone. Once you share your feelings and fears with someone, you may see things a little more clearly. You may be able to deal with problems with greater strength, knowing that you're not alone. Once you're back in control, this fear will disappear.

A FEARLESS SUMMARY

Although many different fears have been discussed in this chapter, we have probably not covered all of the ones you have experienced. In addition, the coping suggestions offered certainly do not include all possible ways of dealing with fear. So what should you do?

You're working on recognizing your fears, right? For some of them, you're modifying your behavior. For others, you're modifying your thinking. Soon you will feel more in control. As this happens, you'll notice your fears begin to diminish. That doesn't mean that they'll all go away. But as you work on them and feel more in control, they'll at least lessen in intensity. You'll feel better knowing that you can do something about some of them, and that you're capable of handling them.

10

Anger

Donna was fed up with joint pain. Practically anyone who went near her received an earful of comments you wouldn't want Mother to hear! Everyone was a victim of this verbal assault—from her doctor to her family. What made her even more angry was that she wanted to slam her fist down on her kitchen table, but she knew it would just make her pain worse. Donna was angry!

In general, people with any restrictive physical conditions may be angry. Because anger results in the build-up of physical energy that needs to be released, it is important for you to learn how to cope with anger.

WHAT IS ANGER?

When you have a desire or goal in mind, and something interferes with your achievement of it, a feeling of tension and hostility may result from the developing frustration. This is what we refer to as anger.

THREE TYPES OF ANGER

It can be helpful to discuss three different ways of experiencing anger. *Rage* is the expression of violent, uncontrolled anger. If Donna was feeling upset about her condition, and a "friend" told her that her joints would still be healthy if she had taken better care of herself, you can imagine how angry she might be. Her anger might even lead her to say or do things that would certainly not enhance the prospects of a long-lasting, warm relationship with this person! Rage is probably the most intense anger you can experience. It is an outward expression of anger, as it results in a visible explosion. Rage can be a destructive release of the intense physical energy that builds up.

A second type of anger is *resentment*. This is the feeling of anger that is usually kept inside. What if Donna listened to her friend's well-meaning comments, smiled and said nothing, but was seething inside? Resentment is a growing, smoldering feeling of anger directed toward a person or an object. However, it is kept bottled up. It tends to sit uncomfortably within you, and can create even more physiological and psychological damage.

The third type of anger is *indignation*. Indignation is considered the most appropriate, positive type of anger. It is released in a more controlled way. If Donna had responded to the comments by stating that she appreciated her friend's concern, but would prefer no advice at this point or she might scream, this might have been a more appropriate response. Obviously, these three types of anger can occur in combination, or in different ways. However, understanding the different ways of experiencing anger can help you to cope with it more effectively.

CAUSES OF ANGER

Obviously, there are lots of things that can make you angry. You may get angry waiting for your doctor to see you. You wouldn't be too thrilled if you had to cancel plans at the last moment. You may get angry if you are told you need yet another type of medication.

Insults from other people, aside from everyday frustrations, can cause anger. "If you didn't play so much tennis, your joints would still be working!" This is not the kind of comment that would make you feel friendly! If you feel that someone is taking advantage of you, or you feel forced to do something that you do not want to do, anger may result. If you do not have the ability or confidence to say "no" when friends ask for a favor, this can create feelings of anger, especially when combined with the fact that you may not feel well.

In addition to the causes of anger mentioned above, there is one more. How about RA as a cause of anger? Aren't you angry about this? There may not be any specific reason you can point to. Or you might be able to list dozens of reasons. But being aware of this is important, because you must be aware of the anger to help yourself deal with it. Unfortunately, resolving your anger won't eliminate the inflammation of RA. Nor should you say that you'll only stop being angry when RA is a thing of the past. Neither attitude will help you. As we go on, we will be discussing ways of reducing anger and feeling better.

Does Your Mind Make You Angry?

It is important to realize that anger exists uniquely in the mind of each angry individual. This anger is a direct result of your thoughts, rather than events. The event by itself does not make you angry. Rather, it leads to your *interpretation* of the event—the way you think or feel about it. That's what can make you angry. This is a very important point, one that will be discussed in much more detail a little bit later in the section, *Dealing With Anger.* Stay tuned. . . .

ANGER AND YOUR BODY

When you are angry, a number of physiological responses occur in your body. Breathing becomes more rapid, blood pressure increases (you may feel like your blood is "boiling"), and your heart may begin to pound. Your face may get "hot," and your muscles become tense. You may feel stronger when angry. The more intense the anger is, the greater this feeling of power. I'm sure you can remember a time when you were so angry that you felt you had superhuman strength.

Anger is a form of energy. The more physical energy that builds up in the body due to anger, the more necessary it becomes for you to release it. The energy cannot be destroyed, so if it is not released in some constructive manner, it will eventually come out in another, less desirable way. Imagine the energy from anger as a stick of dynamite about to explode. If you get rid of it, it will explode away from you. It may cause some damage, but it will not hurt you inside as much as if you swallowed the dynamite to keep others from being hurt. Obviously, the ideal solution is not to throw the stick of dynamite, and not to swallow it, but (are you ready for this?) to try and de-fuse the dynamite! More about de-fusing soon.

Usually, extreme anger can pass quickly. If, however, the anger lasts for a long period of time, it can have physically damaging effects on the body. You've all heard about some of the physical problems that can result from holding in anger: ulcers, hypertension, headaches. Anger can also cause a stress response that may exacerbate your RA. It's just not good for your body.

When anger becomes extreme or turns into rage, you may feel like exploding. You may feel that, unless you are able to punch, kick, or hit something, and get rid of the anger in some way, you may lose control. Hopefully, this angry energy can be released without causing damage to another person, property, or yourself. If, when you finally calm down, you find that you have done something destructive, you may get angry at yourself all over again. Or you may experience another negative emotion, such as guilt.

ANGER AND YOUR MIND

Anger is usually experienced as an unpleasant feeling. However, this unpleasant feeling may exist along with a more pleasant feeling of power or strength. Frequently, the unpleasantness of anger is related to its consequences—knowing what you do when you are angry, and not being happy about it. If you lose control when you're angry, you'll probably even be afraid of it, and of what you might do next time!

DIFFERENT REACTIONS TO ANGER

Maureen, a 28-year-old teacher, was having a hard time with her husband. He was trying to show concern for his wife by not letting her do any housework. But, surprisingly, she *wanted* to clean the house because she believed she felt well enough to do it. His resistance was so persistent, and he was so "saccharin sweet" that Maureen felt it was too much. She wanted to be treated like an adult, able to determine when she could be active. But her husband just wouldn't let up. She was running out of patience. Let's see how this situation might be experienced in different ways.

The "Ignore" Approach

Because you feel like you may completely lose control, or feel overwhelmed by the intensity of your anger, you may try to do whatever you can to avoid the experience. This could include pushing thoughts out of your mind, even when you realize you are getting angry. Maureen might try to get involved in different activities while her husband cleaned the house, and try to ignore the fact that he was being so condescending. Or she might try to agree with everything that he said. Although this might be upsetting, it might at least be temporarily effective in helping her to ignore the smothering. In the long run, however, you can see that this is not the best way to deal with anger.

The "Action" Approach

From another point of view, you might see anger as a necessary part of life, despite its unpleasantness. You know that there will be times when you'll be angry, whether you like it or not. You'll just have to deal with it as best you can.

In this case, Maureen would know that she's not happy being angry, and that she should speak to her husband, to try to get him to understand more about her emotional needs, and how she'd like him to treat her. Hopefully, a better understanding can be reached, but at least Maureen knows that she's doing something about her feelings.

The "Power" Approach

Maybe you enjoy the flow of energy and strength that comes from being angry. You may find that this is when you are best able to assert yourself to accomplish something. Here, Maureen knows that if she is mothered once too often she will explode, and she loves the feeling of power that this anger gives her. She is almost looking forward to the chance to say, "Honey, if you treat me that way once more, I'll take this vacuum cleaner and . . . !" That would wipe the smile off hubby's face!

If you enjoy this feeling, it's possible that you may even provoke situations to make yourself angry! An example of this would be professional football players or boxers, who psyche themselves up before a confrontation with an opponent. For them, becoming as angry as possible is the best preparation for a successful performance.

Your own reaction to anger is unique. It may also change from time to time. There may be times when you accept anger and almost value it as a motivator to accomplish something. At other times you may attempt to push this anger away. Maureen might enjoy expressing her anger. But if she didn't want to cause problems with her husband, upset the rest of the family, or hurt her husband, she might realize that it would be better to have a conversational discussion with him than to shatter his eardrums with her explosion.

IS ANGER GOOD OR BAD?

How can anger possibly be good? Many people feel that nothing constructive can be gained from it. "Avoid anger at all costs," they say, "because nothing good comes from it. . . . Anger will get you into trouble, so don't let it happen." This is true, but only if you don't deal with the anger properly. Anger can be dangerous if it is kept inside. Remember that stick of dynamite? What an explosive example! If anger is released in destructive ways, it can cause problems in relationships (to say the least!). It can create physical problems as well, and can certainly aggravate your RA-related problems. Does this mean that anger can make your condition worse? Well, what if you're so angry at somebody or something that you decide not to take proper care of yourself? For example, you don't take your medication properly, or don't do the prescribed amount of exercise. What if you're angry at someone who cares about you, and normally helps you around the house? That person, if upset by your anger, may be less willing to help you. This may, in turn, make you feel even worse. So if you want your anger to be good instead of bad, try to turn it into something that can be helpful rather than harmful to you.

Anger *can* be constructive. It can mobilize your efforts and make you stronger to deal with an anger-provoking situation. Believe it or not, you might even handle a situation more successfully than you would if you weren't angry! Anger can give you a feeling of power or strength, of confidence or assertiveness. But don't get me wrong. I'm not saying that you should slam your finger with a hammer, or tell someone to punch you, in order to get yourself angry enough to solve all of your problems! What I am saying is that anger can be positive, and it can help you to solve problems. Anger has two main benefits. First, it is an indicator that something is wrong. Something must be creating this feeling of anger—something that needs attention.   Second, anger can motivate you to deal more actively with life's problems. You can become so emotionally charged that it will have a positive effect on your life.

In order for anger to be helpful, there are some very important things to keep in mind. First, don't let yourself become overwhelmed by the anger. Once that happens it is much harder to do what you have to do. Second, don't be afraid of your anger. If you do fear it, you probably won't be able to release it properly. More than likely, it will come out in unhealthy ways, or you'll bottle it up inside. Third, be sure that the way you handle your anger is socially acceptable. Maureen might get a kick out of knocking out her husband's teeth, but would the dentist (or the police) approve? Try to be flexible enough to recognize an appropriate way of releasing your anger.

DEALING WITH ANGER

You've already begun to realize that anger can be constructive. Hopefully, the information you've read so far has been encouraging. But what else can actually be done?

Because anger is such a complex emotion, and because so many things can lead to feelings of anger, there are no simple answers. Sorry about that! Does that mean that there is nothing that anybody can do about anger? No. Some things can be done to reduce the feelings of anger and allow them to be handled more efficiently, comfortably, and safely.

Step One—Admit That You're Angry

The first step in dealing with anger is to recognize that you're angry in the first place. As simple as this may sound, many people cannot even admit when they are angry. They may try to deny it, or rationalize their feelings or behaviors using other explanations. Do you feel that being angry is a sign of weakness? If so, since you don't want to feel weak, you may not even admit that you're angry. You may feel that there is no appropriate reason to be angry, so you're acting in a childish way. But as with anything else, in order to try to change something, you've got to first admit that it exists.

How can you tell that you're angry if you're not sure? (Yes, there are some people who are not sure.) If you feel very tense (jumping at the sound of the telephone), or if you find yourself reacting impulsively (slamming down the phone when you get a wrong number and storming out of the house) or with hostility (cursing at your neighbor for leaving a smidgen of garbage on your lawn), chances are that you're angry. Until you recognize that you are angry, you cannot do anything constructive about it.

Step Two—Where Does Your Anger Come From?

The second step in dealing with anger is trying to identify its source. Where does it come from? What is contributing to it? What events have led to these feelings of anger? Why do you want to break all the furniture? For one thing, your condition may lead to anger. You may be angry with yourself for neglecting your condition. You may feel anger towards your physician, whether justified or not. You may be angry because you have to take so much medication. You may be angry because of the things you can no longer do.

In some cases, the events leading to anger may be quite obvious. In other cases, however, the source of anger may be vague and unclear. It may be hard to pinpoint what is causing it. At such times, you should try to probe even more deeply to come up with possible causes of your anger.

Of course, much of this anger is irrational. But, like other emotional reactions, it must be worked through. It cannot just be pushed away. Simply telling yourself, "Don't be angry," is not enough. You must learn to channel it more effectively.

Guilt can sometimes confuse you if you are trying to identify the source of anger. Josie was a 32-year-old mother of three. She woke up one morning, went downstairs and found her kitchen a disaster area. Taking care of the kitchen was a responsibility that she had given to her children, because she was simply physically unable to handle it. She found herself screaming at them for not fulfilling their responsibilities. In actuality, however, her anger may have been a reflection not of hostility towards her children, but of guilt about her own inability to handle her kitchen responsibilities.

Step Three—Why Are You Angry?

It is now necessary to explain to yourself why you are angry. In Josie's case, she could explain her anger by her inability to do what she wanted to do. Josie wanted to be able to fulfill her responsibilities as a mother and housewife. She felt that taking care of the kitchen was included in this. Because she was unable to do so, she felt angry.

Why is this step important? Mainly, to decide whether or not the anger that you are feeling is realistic. Analyze your reasons for being angry. If you recognize that your reasons are not realistic, this alone can help you to deal with these feelings of anger. If, on the other hand, you can objectively say that your feelings of anger are realistic, then the next step is to decide how you are going to deal with them properly.

How do you deal with them properly? You have already begun! By working through the first three steps, you have received information that will be very helpful in your efforts to deal with your anger.

THOUGHTS CAN MAKE YOU ANGRY

In the past, it was falsely believed that there were only two possible ways to deal with anger: to keep it inside, or to let it out.

But what about a third possibility? Remember before when we talked about de-fusing that stick of dynamite? Our anger is a result of the way we think! In our minds, we are actually interpreting those events that lead to anger. If we can change the way we interpret events, and reorganize our thinking patterns, is it possible to stop creating the anger that we feel? Of course! We can learn to control our thoughts *before* they make us angry, regardless of what the events were. Ask yourself this question: If something happened that made you angry, would everybody in the world be angry because of it? No. The reason why you are angry is because that's the way you think about, or interpret, the event. Other people aren't angry because they did not interpret the event in a way that made them so. For example, let's say you've made a doctor's appointment. Ten minutes before you were ready to leave, the receptionist called to cancel, saying she'd reschedule the appointment at another time. You might be furious, because you felt you should have received more notice, and because you really wanted to be seen. How aggravating!! But others might not interpret it that way, and might not get the least bit angry. So if we can learn to interpret events in a more positive, constructive, and calm manner, we can reduce feelings of anger. We wouldn't have to decide whether we wanted to let anger out or keep it inside because, by controlling our thoughts, anger would not even exist most of the time.

You've already completed one of the first steps in reorganizing your thoughts to prevent anger. You've learned that anger can be good and constructive. It can help you to solve problems, and you don't have to be afraid of it. Just becoming aware of its positive elements can help you to be less afraid of anger. This can help you to deal with the thoughts that may make you angry.

Good Angry Thoughts Vs. Bad Angry Thoughts

Writing down what you think is making you angry can be very helpful. Good angry thoughts can move you to positive, constructive action. You might want to plan your strategies for resolving the problem. On the other hand, many of your thoughts may include so much anger, and be so destructive, that you feel like banging your head against the wall. Be honest when writing down your thoughts, regardless of how violent or profane they may be. Such rich, colorful language can be helpful in getting your feelings out and down on paper. This will ultimately help you to control your anger. Try to look at these thoughts more objectively, the way someone else might look at them. Attempt to bring them down to a more manageable level.

Mental Movies

An interesting technique that can be helpful in controlling anger is imagery, or "watching movies in your mind." When you become angry, you frequently have all kinds of pictures in your head of what is making you angry and what you'd like to do to deal with it. These movies can be very helpful.

For example, imagine that you are very, very tired. Your friend calls to tell you that her car has broken down. Could you please pick up her dry-cleaning? When you tell her that you are too tired to go, she says something about how she can never depend on you for anything. This is a friend? You are furious. At that moment, imagine all the abusive things that you would like to say to her, and imagine the shocked expression on her face. If you ask her to hold on for a moment, and close your eyes and imagine this as if you were actually doing it, you'll probably be able to complete the phone call without destroying a friendship. You may even smile or laugh as you think about the scenes that are playing through your mind. More about imagery in the chapter, *Pain*.

Nora was quite fed up with her son, Pesty Pete. Whenever she asked for his help with normal household chores, his answers were fresh and abusive. Just before she was about to give him a haircut with a meat cleaver, she remembered the mental movie technique. She imagined herself strangling him—his eyeballs popping and gurgling sounds coming from his throat. This helped to get rid of the intense, angry feelings that were making her crazy, and allowed her to deal with Pete more constructively. (No, she's not in jail.)

The Big, Red Stop Sign

Another technique that can help you to control anger is referred to as "thought stopping." Remember: It is the thoughts in your mind that are making you angry. These are the thoughts you have upon interpreting an event. When you find that angry thoughts have come into your head, picture a big red stop sign. Seeing that word in your mind will serve as a momentary distraction. Then concentrate on something you enjoy, whether it is a peaceful, relaxing scene, a type of food that you like to eat, an activity that you enjoy, or a movie or television program. Whatever you choose, you will divert your thinking, and have a better chance of dissipating your anger. You could also participate in a pleasant distracting activity, such as reading a book, taking a walk, or calling a friend, which will also help you to feel less angry.

Change Your Requirements

People often get angry when they want certain things to occur in certain ways. When your specific requirements are not met, you may feel angry. Trying to modify your requirements can help you to cope with anger.

Let's say that you're not feeling well and you decide to call your doctor. The answering service tells you that he is not in the office and that you should get a return call within a half-hour. After forty-five minutes, when he still hasn't returned your call, you are fuming. Why? Because your requirement of a call-back within thirty minutes has not been met. Revise your requirement. Tell yourself that you would have liked a call within thirty minutes, but your doctor may be tied up on another cause, or in transit, or unable to get to a phone. You'll be satisfied if you get a call at his earliest convenience. By modifying the requirement, you can feel less angry.

Another way to benefit from this technique is to write down those thoughts indicating what your requirements are. Then try to write down new, more flexible desires. This will make you feel better.

PUT YOURSELF IN THEIR SHOES

One of the best ways of dealing with anger towards somebody else is to try to understand exactly what that person is feeling: what the person wants, why the person is saying what he or she is saying. This will make you more aware of why somebody else is behaving or talking the way he or she is, and you will be better able to deal with it constructively. This will also help you to understand what the other person will feel if he or she is the target of your abusive release of anger.

LET IT OUT LESS EXPLOSIVELY

We have discussed a number of ways to control your thinking and improve your ability to interpret events in ways that will not allow anger to develop. But what if this doesn't always work? What if there are times when you remain as angry as you were before? What can be done to deal with anger constructively when it already exists?

Talk, Don't Bite

Obviously, it is much more desirable to have a constructive discussion over an issue than an angry exchange of heated words which accomplishes nothing. In most cases, anger arises from a conflict or problem with another person. Therefore, it is frequently helpful to improve your ability to get your point across constructively. You are trying to negotiate a better resolution to a problem that may exist between you and somebody else. A heated argument, or "fighting fire with fire," is not the answer. Instead, you want to fight the fire by dousing it—reducing the heatedness of the argument. Try complimenting the person or looking for the positive things in what that person is saying to you, even if you're angry. This works in two ways.

One, it will probably surprise the person. Two, you'll be focusing on words or thoughts that are more constructive, rather than letting yourself get angry because of what's being said. Calmly restate your feelings.

How About Physical Activity?

In general, one of the best outlets for releasing angry energy is physical activity. Because of RA, though, this outlet may not be as available as you'd like. Interestingly, it has been found that physical energy from anger can be released by watching things. For example, by watching a sporting event, you aren't releasing energy through participation in the sport, but you may still be able to "get into it" and reduce your anger that way. Or try watching a particularly violent or emotionally draining movie. You can become so totally absorbed that the energy building up from anger is released through worry, fear, or excitement. A movie or book that allows you to identify with the characters, or where the characters allow release of anger, can be beneficial as well. A common and very effective outlet for anger, especially among children, is crying. I'm sure you've heard of the therapeutic effects of a good cry. However, this technique is not for everyone. People who can be more open in expressing their emotions may be better able to benefit from this outlet.

Some people like to count to ten when angry. This can distract you from what is making you angry, giving you a chance to calm down and think about it more constructively. Try counting to a thousand, if necessary!

LET US REVIEW

It is very important to remember that events alone do not make you angry. It is your thoughts, your interpretations of these events, that lead to anger. Even if something really terrible happens, it is the meaning that you give to this particular event that makes you angry. It is the way you think about this terrible event that creates your anger. Since your thinking makes you angry, *you* are responsible for feeling this way. Therefore, you can be just as responsible for changing your thinking to help yourself cope with anger, or at least reducing it to a more manageable level.

The best way to handle anger is probably to be in control enough so that it doesn't build up in the first place. But if it does, remember that if anger is channeled and used constructively, it does have its benefits. Uncontrolled anger can be an unpleasant, negative, destructive emotion. Your efforts are best spent in trying to figure out how to reorganize your thinking so that it doesn't get out of hand.

11

Guilt

Have you ever felt guilty? Many individuals with RA say that they have. Guilt is a very unpleasant emotion. Take the case of Yolanda, a 32-year-old mother of two. She was very unhappy because she couldn't be the kind of mother she wanted to be. Why not? Well, because she just couldn't participate in enough activities with her kids. So having RA made her feel guilty that she was being a bad mother. Hard to cope? You bet! Let's take a look at what leads to guilty feelings.

THE TWO COMPONENTS OF GUILT

Feelings of guilt usually have two components. The first of these is the "wrongdoing;" you feel that you have either done something wrong, or haven't done something that you should have done. The second component is the "self-blame;" you blame yourself for doing this wrong thing, and feel that you are "bad" because of it. That's the culprit! It is the concept of "badness" that creates the guilty feeling. If you *feel* bad about doing something wrong, this is normal and understandable. But when you start telling yourself that you *are* bad, guilt follows. What if other people tell you that "it's o.k.?" This may not help. Your feeling of guilt may have nothing to do with what others tell you or what they think. Even if they disagree with you, these are still your feelings. Remember: Your guilt comes from the feeling that you are a bad person, rather than from feeling bad about what you have done. Is it fitting to label yourself as a bad person or blame yourself because you've done something wrong? Even if you have done something wrong, it's better to label that particular behavior as bad, rather than yourself.

Is the behavior that you are blaming yourself for really that terrible or wrong? Does it justify the feeling of badness that leads to guilt? In Yolanda's case, then, she felt guilty because of her RA. Does that make sense? Did she make it happen? Of course not. Yolanda might feel better, therefore, if she emphasized the *quality* of time spent with her children, rather than the *quantity*.

WHAT IS VS. WHAT OUGHT TO BE

Guilt feelings about the inability to handle children or the lack of time to spend with children are very common for mothers with RA. On the other hand, men tend to feel more guilty about the inability to advance in their careers or to fulfill their job responsibilities the way they feel they should. How about Phil, a 52-year-old husband and father of two? He felt guilty because he was not able to work as hard at his job as he used to. He therefore earned less money—not enough to provide all of the luxuries he and his family would have enjoyed. Feeling under pressure, Phil tried to work harder to earn more money, which in turn made him feel worse physically. This created the guilty feelings. He felt less capable of being the bread-winner in the family, and was therefore a bad father and husband. How does one cope with these feelings?

Do you see a difference between the way you are doing something and the way you think you should be doing it? If so, you can really feel the old guilt horns! How do you work this out? Major union/ management problems would be easier to solve! Can you work harder or do more? If you can, then do it. If not, try examining your day-to-day goals for working and living. Check to see if these goals are practical, considering what you can and cannot do because of your RA. Try to take more pride in what you *can* do. Although most people hate hearing, "things could be worse," this phrase is quite true. You might not be able to do anything at all. If you concentrate on the things you can do, and place less emphasis on what you can't, your feelings of guilt will diminish. You'll feel a lot better. Changing the emphasis in your thinking will also help you to lessen the gap between what is and what ought to be. This is what led to these guilty feelings in the first place.

Does this approach work only for working men? No. It applies to anyone who feels guilty because of falling short of expectations and desires. Milly, a 16-year-old student, was feeling guilty because she was unable to devote the amount of time to her schoolwork as she previously had, or as she would have liked. She was more and more reluctant to go to school because she was so frequently unprepared, and she missed a number of school days because of RA. The guilt she felt affected her schoolwork even more. How might Milly cope with these guilty feelings? It might be beneficial for Milly to speak to each of her teachers and explain how RA was affecting her, cautioning her teachers that physical problems might restrict her from devoting the same amount of time to her schoolwork as she had previously, and that her attendance might not be as good as it had been. At that point, it would be helpful to discuss possible methods for making up for this, such as extra projects that she might be able to work on when she was feeling up to it, or alternate arrangements for testing (to try to show her teachers that even with less time available for studying she was still interested in succeeding in class). By working with her teachers and setting more realistic goals, the feelings of guilt related to having RA and its effect on her schoolwork should decrease.

TALK IT OVER

It is very important to discuss how you feel about your condition with others who may be affected by it. It is helpful to talk over feelings with the important people in your life, to share concerns, and try to figure out solutions to problems. Jill, a 46-year-old woman who had been married for 20 years, had enjoyed a very active social life before developing rheumatoid arthritis. In addition to going out on weekends, she and her husband would play tennis with friends or participate in other social activities at least two or three evenings during the week. Now, because of the pain and fatigue she was experiencing from RA, she had to restrict her activities. She just couldn't go out as frequently. She couldn't even play tennis at all. Sometimes, she wouldn't want to go out even once during an entire week. Not only did she feel unhappy about her condition, but she felt extremely guilty at holding her husband back. She felt that he couldn't have a good time because of her. It would be helpful for Jill to discuss alternatives with her husband. Arriving at a solution, with her husband's cooperation, could effectively reduce guilt feelings and improve the marriage.

THOUGHTS CAN HURT, TOO

So far, we have been discussing how doing the wrong thing can lead to guilt. But it's not only "behavioral mistakes" that can lead to guilty feelings. Thoughts can also become upsetting enough to lead to guilt.

Sometimes, you may feel guilty without doing anything wrong. You may be merely thinking things that cause guilt. Pam, a 29-year-old mother of three young children, was feeling terribly guilty. Why? Her 30-year-old husband was spending many hours taking care of the kids and helping her with the housework. Pam knew that her condition meant that she couldn't do what she used to, but she felt bad because her husband had to do so much. She was afraid that he would eventually start complaining. Should Pam blame herself and feel guilty because of her condition—something she could not control? Since she hadn't really done anything wrong, Pam would feel better if she modified her thinking.

In order to successfully cope with guilt, you must first focus on what led to the guilty feelings. Have you actually done something wrong? Have you really neglected something you shouldn't have? You may feel guilty about your thoughts or desires, rather than specific actions or behaviors. Recognize that, if you haven't done anything to lead to guilt, then you should identify those thoughts that are making you feel like a bad person. Change them. If you can learn to talk to yourself in a positive way, looking at your thoughts objectively and constructively, guilt can be reduced.

Frequently, as in Pam's case, feeling guilty is related to seeing yourself as responsible for others' actions or behaviors. The more responsible you feel, the more guilt you may feel, especially if you cannot fulfill your responsibility. Frequently, just asking the question "why?" will point out that this thinking is unrealistic. That alone can help to reduce guilt. This is another reason why discussions with other important people are helpful. They may explain why taking the responsibility for someone else is inappropriate. Be sure to place feelings of responsibility in proper perspective. There is a limit as to how responsible you should feel for others' actions or feelings. Nor are you responsible for having RA, and for any restrictions this may place on you. Pam should recognize that nobody was forcing her husband to take over household responsibilities. He chose this course of action. Pam would have less guilt if she didn't feel responsible for her husband's choice. Realize that when individuals are not forced into an activity, they participate out of choice and desire. The same holds true for this book. You *are* reading it out of choice and desire, aren't you?

"SHOULD" THOUGHTS

Among the most common causes of guilt are thoughts containing the word "should." "Should" is a dirty word! Examples of such thoughts are, "I should have been able to finish that job today. . . . We should have that party; all our friends have entertained us this year. . . . You should have let me do the dishes . . . I shouldn't have any more pain." These "should" thoughts imply that you must be just about perfect, and on top of everything. When there is a difference between what you feel should occur and what actually does occur, guilt can result. You will become upset whenever you fall short of your "should." Should thoughts lead to guilt simply because they are not sensible, realistic, or justifiable? Should you blame yourself because the thoughts determine goals that you may not be able to fulfill?

Now that I've explained what you *shouldn't* do, what exactly *should* you do? In order to feel better and reduce feelings of guilt, it is helpful to reword your thoughts to eliminate "should" thoughts. Try to use less demanding words. Say, "It would be nice if I could finish that job today, but I can't," rather than, "I should finish that job today." If your physical condition is restricting your activities, you'll feel much more guilty when "should" thoughts remind you of unfulfilled obligations. If you have trouble changing the wording of your "should" thoughts, try asking yourself, "Why should I . . . ?" or "Who says I should . . . ?" or "Where is it written that I should. . . . ?" This may help you decide whether you are setting up impossible requirements for yourself. It can also help you to reduce your feelings of guilt.

Let's say, for example, that you are thinking of having a party because all your friends have invited you to get-togethers. Ask yourself why you should. Is it because the "Party Rulebook" tells you that, if you don't have a party, your friendship license will be revoked? Is it because, if you don't have a party, your friends (some friends!) won't invite you to their homes anymore? As you think about the realistic answers to these questions, it will be easier to realize that you don't have to have a party. Although it would be nice, it is more acceptable to wait until you feel better.

THE CONSEQUENCES OF GUILT

So far, we've been discussing what leads to guilt, how you may feel, and how you can try to adjust your thoughts and behaviors to feel better. But what happens if you have not yet been successful in eliminating guilt? People who feel guilty frequently act in negative ways to hide from these feelings. There may be a tendency to indulge in "escape" behaviors, such as drinking or excessive sleeping, which do not deal with problems head-on but, instead, attempt to push them away.

Ruth, a 58-year-old bookkeeper, felt guilty because she had stopped making plans with her friends. She did this because she was embarrassed about how many times she had to cancel plans at the last minute. As a result, she began to lose friends, and her guilt became more and more difficult to bear. She began drinking each day, and going to bed right after dinner, in an attempt to "escape" and forget her misery. This behavior did not help the situation any, and it certainly didn't help her medical condition. In fact, it was downright dangerous. Not only did it compound the problem, but there was the added danger of mixing alcohol and medication. Now Ruth had something else to feel guilty about: her escape behavior. This could increase the feeling of badness, leading to even more guilt and creating a vicious cycle.

The first step towards improvement is to look past the escape behavior and identify whatever is causing the guilt. Consider what can be done to rectify the problem causing the guilt. At the same time, try to eliminate any escape behavior, recognizing that it is only a cop-out. It is possible, however, for there to be no clear-cut solution to the events or feelings creating guilt. If, for example, Ruth's physical condition is keeping her from making plans with her friends, can she believe that the only way to make things better is for her to force herself to do things she physically shouldn't? That would be ridiculous. Don't give up because no complete solutions exist. Look for partial solutions, which can still help to reduce guilt by reminding you that you are trying to improve the situation. Ruth's RA won't go away, but she could at least try to reduce her reluctance to get together with friends. And, she certainly could try to explain the problem to her friends so she'd be less embarrassed if she does have to cancel plans.

OTHER SUGGESTIONS

We've talked a lot about how thoughts and behaviors can cause guilt. But what if you just feel guilty and can't remember what you were thinking or doing to make you feel that way? How can you start using all these great thought-changing ideas if you don't remember what thoughts you want to change? Good question! In order to identify those "target" thoughts or behaviors, you might want to keep a brief, written log of feelings or activities that may have caused your guilt. Once you have written these things down, you can then begin figuring out how to change them, improving your outlook, and reducing your guilt.

Beth, age 35, had been feeling increasingly guilty recently but didn't really know why. By keeping a log, she noticed that she had been arriving at work late on a regular basis. She wasn't aware of how frequently she had been late, and she had always been proud of her punctuality. The log helped her to see that she must give herself more time to get "loose" in the morning in order to be more punctual. As she worked on this problem, her guilt lessened.

What about those negative thoughts that lead to guilt? It can be very helpful to try and turn these thoughts around, making them more positive and guilt-free. For example, let's say that you feel guilty because you believe you are a bad parent. Ask yourself if you have ever done anything that a good parent might do. Just about every parent can come up with something. This starts the process of eliminating your "bad parent blues." The idea is to turn your mind's negative thoughts into reasonable, positive ones. This way, the feeling of guilt won't take a strangle-hold!

A FINAL GUILTY THOUGHT

Guilt is a very destructive emotion—one that can certainly interfere with your success in coping with rheumatoid arthritis. By becoming aware of how guilt develops, you have a much better chance of effectively employing coping strategies to reduce guilt and its negative effects.

12

Stress

What is stress? Stress is a response that occurs in your body. It helps you mobilize your strength to deal with different things happening in your life. Many things occur each day that require you to adapt. These are the "stressors." All the changes that occur in your body when something (the stressor) provokes you are known as the "stress response."

With rheumatoid arthritis, you may experience stress for many reasons. For example, pain alone can cause stress. Your concern about whether your disease will get worse can cause stress. Worries about joint replacement surgery can be stressful. Problems with medication are also stressors. Any one of these—and more—can provoke the stress response.

IS STRESS GOOD OR BAD?

A certain amount of stress is normal—and necessary. Stress helps you to "get your act together," and prepares you to handle your life in the best possible way. Now you're probably thinking, "So why do I always hear people talking about how stress can be harmful?" When people talk about the harmful effects of stress, they are referring to situations where there is *too much* stress. Then it can become destructive. If left unchecked, it can eat away at you and drain all of your energy.

Reasonable amounts of stress can be handled. In fact, they can even be helpful. This chapter, however, is concerned with harmful stress—the kind that can hurt if not controlled. The word "stress" is used very frequently these days. It describes those things that create nervousness, anxiety, tension, anger, or an upset feeling. Actually, these are all parts of stress, rather than the same thing. In other words, they may cause the stress response.

Fran, a 35-year-old housewife, was under pressure. Her husband was bringing his boss home for dinner. Because she knew she got exhausted easily, she carefully paced herself as she prepared the meal so she wouldn't get run down. The stress she felt was tolerable; that is, until the phone rang. Her husband called telling her that, due to an emergency business meeting that evening, they'd be arriving two hours early! Fran's stress was no longer tolerable!

WHO FEELS STRESS?

Everyone experiences stress. Nobody escapes it. But since stress can be positive or negative, learning how to respond positively will lead to a more successful emotional and physical life. If you have a hard time responding to stress, this won't be easy. Some people are more vulnerable to negative stress responses than others. Are you?

THE STRESS RESPONSE

Every person has a unique way of responding to stress. Stress control management (effectively managing the way you respond to stress) is within your reach. Your pattern of response depends on a number of things—your upbringing, self-esteem, beliefs about yourself and the world, what you say to yourself, and how you guide yourself in your thoughts and actions. The degree to which you feel in control of your life plays a role in your stress response. The way you feel physically and emotionally, and the way you get along with people, are also a part of it. To sum it up, everyone's method of dealing with stress is unique and individual, and depends on a complex combination of thoughts and behaviors.

Stressor + Interpretation = Stress Response

The way that you respond to stress depends on the "chemistry" between two factors. The first factor is the stressor, or the outside pressures. What is going on around you that is creating the reactions? The second factor is what is within you, or how you interpret things. It is the interaction of the stimulus and your own internal reaction that determines your response to stress. (Sound familiar? Yes, it's the same "formula" that can be applied to anger, depression, and all the other emotions.) This equation has important implications for coping with stress, when you realize that it isn't just the environment that causes your response, but also the way you interpret the stressor. Some stressors in the environment would produce stress in anybody. What would happen, for example, if somebody pointed a knife at your throat? Calm acceptance, or a stress response? Get the point? It's important to learn how to reduce the number of stressors that negatively affect you, and improve your reaction to those you can't avoid.

Body Vs. Mind

How do you respond to stress? Like one's response to anger or other mobilizing emotions, there are two main ways: physically and cognitively. A cognitive response includes the way you think and feel. Most people respond to stress in both ways, although it is possible for you to respond in only one way.

What happens physically? If you experience a stressful situation, the circulatory system speeds up. Blood is pushed rapidly towards different parts of the body, particularly those parts necessary to protect you. Because the blood supply is diverted towards these essential parts, the supply to the digestive system is usually reduced. As a result, the digestive process slows down, making it work less efficiently.

Chronic or prolonged stress puts a severe strain on your body. When your body is strong, it can fight off most foreign invaders, bacteria, and germs. As a result, many diseases can be avoided. But prolonged stress puts such a strain on the body that your defense mechanisms may break down. This, in turn, makes your body more vulnerable to the very problems you'd like to avoid!

Have you heard of the "fight or flight" syndrome? Animals do this when they feel threatened. The animal prepares either to fight or run away, a purely physical response. You will not see an animal standing there, scratching his head, and thinking about what should be done! But humans have the unique ability to think and reason! Lucky us! So we include cognitive responses in our repertoire. (By the way, researchers feel that this is one of the main reasons why human beings are susceptible to so much stress-related physical illness. By thinking, instead of acting, we may not be dealing with stress as effectively as we might.)

When does stress lead to physical problems? When you can't respond to stress in a way that eliminates it, the stress continues unabated. Being unable to do anything about it may cause even more stress, creating a vicious cycle. This can take its toll on your body.

You may be vulnerable to stress in your own unique way. Certain parts of your body may tend to be more vulnerable and, when stressors occur, it is these parts that feel the effect. For example, have you ever felt extreme intestinal discomfort and automatically clutched your stomach because of stress? Or have you ever endured a painful headache? Stress may have even played a role in RA, or in another illness or condition that you've suffered.

What happens if you respond to stress physically? You may tremble or perspire. Your face may flush. You may feel a surge of adrenaline flowing through your body. Your mouth may become dry or you may feel nauseous. Your breathing may become more rapid and shallow. Your heart may begin to pound. Your muscles may become tight, creating headaches, cramps, or other painful reactions. Sounds lovely, doesn't it?

Your cognitive or emotional response to stress may not be as visible. You may not be able to concentrate as well. Your attention span may be reduced. You may have trouble learning something new. You may be afraid to do things. You may withdraw or feel nervous. You may lose confidence in yourself. You'll become aware of any unpleasant physical responses, and this may make you feel even more stressed. For example, if you feel stress and respond with shallow, rapid breathing or heart palpitations, being aware of these physical responses may create even more stress. This can lead to feelings of panic.

THREE RESPONSES TO STRESS

When a stressful stimulus occurs, you will most likely respond in one of three ways. You might respond immediately and impulsively without giving enough thought to a better response. You might not respond at all, and either try to ride it out, or become so frozen that you are unable to respond. Finally, you may respond to stressors in a well-planned, organized, and effective manner. If so, you may not even need this chapter! But if not, read on!

HOW TO DEAL WITH STRESS

Remember: Stress can be managed and controlled, but it cannot be eliminated. Stress will always exist. You can deal with the amount of stress you endure and how intense that stress may be, but you'll never be able to make it go away. For a person with RA, it is especially important that stress be controlled. Why? Although stress by itself does not cause RA, it can certainly play a major role in exacerbating your RA symptoms.

Let's begin by mentioning the wrong ways of responding to stress. These are the ways that *don't* help you: smoking, getting drunk, using drugs, overeating, and overactivity. Not only will these activities distract you or delay the effects of stress, but they can also hurt you.

So what should you do? Try to learn new, more appropriate ways of dealing with stress than the methods you've been using.

Relaxation Procedures

The best way to start controlling stress is by using relaxation procedures. Try the "quick release" method discussed in the introductory chapter of this section. Other successful methods of relaxation include meditation, self-hypnosis, imagery, or even a warm shower! Deep breathing alone can help to eliminate tension from the body, slow down the heart, and create a better sense of well-being. Learning to relax can be helpful in reducing the amount of stress you are experiencing. It will give your body a chance to rest and recuperate as well. A stronger body can deal more effectively with the ravages of stress (or of life)! Relaxation will also help you to sleep better. Have you been experiencing any sleep problems since the onset of your condition???

Pinpointing Stressors

Stress is a type of energy that needs release. It can be handled either positively or negatively. Stress is negative when you cannot handle it well. In order to learn how to cope successfully, you must first identify your stressors. What, specifically, is causing you to feel stress? Maybe you're concerned about medication. Maybe you fear surgery. Maybe you're just having a hard time with pain or other symptoms of rheumatoid arthritis. These are all possible RA-related stressors and, of course, there are plenty more.

What if you're not sure what's causing it? How can you figure out what it is? One way is to keep a record of your activities and experiences, using numerical ratings, such as a scale called the SUD Scale. SUD stands for Subjective Units of Disturbance. How does it work? Ratings on this scale range from 0 to 100, depending on the amount of stress you're experiencing. Use 100 to represent the most extreme and disturbing stress, and 0 to represent no stress (total and complete relaxation). Then rate your activities and experiences on the SUD scale. The ones with the higher SUD numbers are the ones causing you the most stress. For example, loud, blasting music from your teenager's radio might be rated a whopping 85!

Identify Your Stress Reactions

Once you have begun identifying your stressors, you must then become completely aware of your responses to them. Are they more physiological or psychological? What parts of your body seem to be the most vulnerable? What kind of reactions does your body show? Does your attention span suffer? Do you start losing confidence, or feel like you're slipping? As you become more aware of this, you will develop a more complete picture of your unique stress response. You'll be able to recognize the stressors that affect you and how you react to them. You'll then be better able to decide whether or not you should modify your behavior in responding to the stressor.

What's the next step? Once you recognize which stressors are negative, try to determine whether or not you can eliminate them. If you can, start figuring out how to do it. Removing the source of stress is an obvious and logical way to manage stress. Develop a plan of attack. This might include a number of alternate strategies, all designed to remove or minimize the impact of the stressor. Taking a sledge hammer to that radio might be great, if you could lift the hammer!

But what happens if you can't eliminate the source of your stress? You'll then have to work on your means of interpreting what's going on. You'll have to work on your thinking, and your responding, in order to manage stress. In such cases, changing the stressor is out of your control, but changing the way you react isn't. You might want to use some of the suggestions discussed in the chapters, *Depression* and *Anger*. The use of *systematic desensitization*, discussed in the chapter, *Fears and Anxieties*, can also be beneficial. Many techniques for changing your thinking have already been discussed in previous chapters.

Physical Stress Relievers

Certain physical activities can be great for stress control. For example, some people can relieve tension or stress by driving. As long as the driver continues to observe safety rules, driving can be very relaxing.

Exercise

Another important way of dealing with stress is by exercising. As you'll read later, exercise is not only important in helping you deal with stress, it is one of the most essential components of your treatment program for RA. Regardless of how RA is affecting you, there are still exercises you can do to help yourself control stress. Virtually any type of exercise can be effective. Anything that gets the body moving, gets the heart pumping faster, and allows for a release of tension, is ideal.

Keeping Busy—The Fun Way

Hobbies or other leisure activities can be very helpful. They can divert your attention away from the stressful situation, directing it towards something more enjoyable. These activities will also help you feel productive. A lack of productivity may be one of the stressors giving you problems in the first place!

Another technique for dealing with stress is sleep. Some people have difficulty sleeping when experiencing high levels of stress. However, cat naps, short naps, or even prolonged periods of sleep may be possible and can help reduce stress.

IN CONCLUSION

What are your goals? If stress is interfering with your achievement of these goals, then your stress response is negative. Learning how to control stress is a very necessary part of successfully achieving your goals, as well as successfully coping with rheumatoid arthritis.

13

Other Emotions

The emotions we've covered so far in this section are not the only ones, of course. Worry, for example, is a basic emotion. What might you worry about? Have you got a month to discuss all the possibilities? You've probably worried about the future, what your life will be like, whether you should have a joint replaced, how life will change because of rheumatoid arthritis, among countless other things. What other emotions enter into the picture? This chapter will discuss four other emotions common in life with RA: boredom, envy, loneliness, and upset.

BOREDOM

Hopefully, by this time, you are not so bored that you have stopped reading! As long as you aren't bored, let's talk a little about boredom! What an empty feeling! It's one of the worst feelings anyone can experience. It has been said that more problems and serious tragedies come from being bored than from any other single condition.

Why are you bored? There may be no meaningful activity going on, no stimulation or excitement. Your life may seem to be going nowhere. Nothing is challenging you, and there's no incentive to do anything. Because you weren't born bored, you must have learned to be bored. You weren't always bored, and even now you are not always bored. There are still certain things that hold your attention from time to time. Right?

Is Rheumatoid Arthritis Boring?

I bet you never thought of rheumatoid arthritis as boring. But it can be, primarily because of any restrictions your condition may impose on you. Many activities that provided enjoyment for you in the past may now be out of reach.

Olive hated the fact that her condition prevented her from knitting. She was tired of music, and she didn't want to read. Was Olive bored? Definitely! But did she *have* to be bored? No! Her family and friends suggested that she try new activities, and Olive was soon able to feel less bored.

So what should you do? Don't let your condition cause you to give up on life. Distinguish between what you can do and what you can't. If you do have to curtail any activities because of rheumatoid arthritis, you'll do so. If you have to drop an activity, you'll drop it. But you don't have to eliminate all activities from your life simply because you feel you won't complete them.

"Unboring" Yourself

What can you do about it? The first step is to analyze why you are bored. What is causing the boredom? Obviously, figuring this out will help you to determine how you can improve things. Then you'll want to see what you can do to add some interest to your life. But don't feel that you must push yourself to enjoy something. Forcing yourself to become amused rarely works. You may find that activities you used to enjoy have become artificial and uninteresting. You may no longer get any pleasure from them. That doesn't mean, however, that you should give up, and not try to do anything. You do want to try some new activities that will make your life more interesting. Don't limit yourself to those things that used to interest you. Preferences change. Try things that never interested you before, because maybe now they will spark an interest in you.

Learn Something New!

One of the most effective weapons against boredom is learning. The mind is like a sponge, always ready and willing to soak up more information and knowledge. Select a potentially interesting topic you don't know much about. Try to learn something about it. You may want to begin by simply going to the library and reading some books on the topic. Maybe you'd like to enroll in an adult education course. Often, boredom quickly disappears once you are involved in something new. Learning is a great way to do this.

You can also become bored if your social life is not the greatest. What can you do about this? Once again, try to learn something, especially by taking courses of some kind. Aside from the mental stimulation you'll get from such learning activities, you may also meet interesting and challenging people. Increasing your circle of friends is a good way to fight boredom.

Anticipation!

One of the best ways to fight boredom is to always give yourself something to look forward to. It doesn't matter how small this may be. It can be as simple as reading a chapter of a good book, writing a letter, making that phone call you've been looking forward to, watching a television program you've been excited about, or meeting somebody special for lunch. Try to schedule something to look forward to every day. This way, even if part of your day seems boring, whether you're doing menial chores or just resting to build up your strength, you will at least have something enjoyable to look forward to. You won't give the weeds of boredom a chance to take root!

Goal-Setting

Set goals for yourself, both short-term and long-term. Boredom can arise from plodding along with no purpose in life. Having something specific and tangible to shoot for can be helpful in fighting boredom. This doesn't mean you'll never be bored. You may still have to give yourself an occasional kick in the derriere to keep moving toward those goals. But isn't it better to have something to shoot for than to have nothing at all?

ENVY

You've heard the cliche, "The grass is always greener. . . ." If you have RA, you are probably envious of others who do not. This is understandable. You may even be envious of other people's joints!

Envy can be a destructive emotion, because it's a type of self-torture. It can be very painful. You're constantly putting yourself down and comparing yourself with the better qualities of somebody else. You feel inferior. This can lead to other feelings as well, such as anger or depression.

Why is envy a problem? Because it shows that you are not satisfied with being yourself. You want to be like somebody else. You want to have what somebody else has. Does this mean that the other person has a happy life? Is that person happier than you in every way? You may have rheumatoid arthritis, but this doesn't mean that everything else about the other person's life is superior. Stop and think for a moment. I'm sure you can come up with some areas in which your life is better!

Is Envy a Positive Emotion?

In general, emotions usually serve a purpose. Emotions such as anger and anxiety mobilize you to prepare to handle their sources. On the other hand, envy is a destructive emotion. It does not have the positive qualities that other emotions may have. But maybe you can find something positive in envy. If you recognize that you're envious, analyze the reasons why. Try to change this by concentrating on yourself and your own attributes. Don't let envy get you down.

How Does Envy Occur?

Basically, there are four conditions necessary for you to feel envy. First, you feel deprived. You feel like you can't have something that you want or need. This doesn't just mean money, pleasure, working joints, or even health. Envy is an intense feeling that involves more than this. It seems like your feeling of need lies deep inside. Second, somebody else has whatever it is that you feel you're missing. Third, you feel powerless to do anything about it. You feel totally unable to change the circumstances that have made you envious in the first place. This helplessness causes you to feel more and more bitter. This makes you even more envious! Fourth, there is a change in the relationship between you and whatever it is that you envy, be it person, object, or situation. You no longer simply compare yourself with the other, but feel fiercely competitive. You may begin to feel that the only reason you don't have what you would like is because somebody else does.

If you feel envious, is it necessarily the same kind of envy that everyone feels? No. There are actually two types of envy. One is an envy of tangible things (cars, boats, homes, friends, and so on). The other is less tangible, such as pleasure or health. If you have RA, you may still have many tangible things. You may still have a family, a car, and a place to live. You may still have a job. But the fact that you're not happy with your medical condition makes you envious, and this is more emotional.

What Can You Do?

Concentrate on being yourself. Increase the positive benefits and enjoyments you can get out of life. Why worry about comparing yourself with somebody else? What's that going to do? Sure, your body may not be functioning the way it used to. But that doesn't mean you can't enjoy life as much as somebody else can. Set up reasonable goals for yourself, considering other things you have and how you feel. Then you can say that you're living your life as enjoyably as anybody else. This is more possible when you do not compare yourself with somebody else. Remember, you are you. Concentrate on making the best of your own life.

LONELINESS

There is a difference between being alone and being lonely. Being alone simply means that there is no one else with you. This can be either good or bad. But being lonely is usually a downer. If you feel lonely, it doesn't really matter whether or not there's anyone with you. What's more important is where you stand with other people. Loneliness is a sad, empty feeling, but one that is usually created by you.

Why might you feel lonely? You may feel left out if you can't spend time with others the way you used to, either because you're not feeling well or you can't do what others want to do. Maybe you feel lonely because other people don't want to be with you. You may decide to change some of your relationships because you don't want to take a chance of being rejected. Does that mean you're happy about these changes? No.

It's hard to be lonely. Not just because you feel bad, though. It actually takes effort to make yourself lonely—it doesn't just happen. And you have to work hard to keep yourself feeling lonely. There are many opportunities to be with people. As result, loneliness usually occurs out of choice rather than accident. In order to be really lonely, you'd have to purposely exclude everyone around you from your life. You'd have to always be on your guard, protecting yourself from the horrible possibility of making a new friend!

Why Be Lonely?

Why might you want to be lonely? There are four reasons. First, if you're lonely, you probably enjoy being lonely. This may contradict what you complain about to everyone else. If you're lonely, it's because you like it enough not to do anything about it. Second, if you're lonely, it's because you're hard to please. You may feel that you don't want to even bother trying to create new relationships because no one meets all of your requirements. Third, if you're lonely it may be because you feel you must be lonely. You've resigned yourself to it. You tell yourself that this is part of the price you have to pay for having RA! Fourth, and probably most important, if you're lonely it may be because you're scared. You're afraid to develop new relationships. You're afraid to make yourself vulnerable because you're afraid of being rejected. You may recall previous experiences that did not work out the way you wanted. You don't want to relive the hurt and pain.

Break Your Lonely Ways

Reading about this isn't easy, especially if you are a lonely person. Why? It's not easy to think that maybe you did this to yourself! But there is still a light at the end of the tunnel! Recognize where your feelings of loneliness come from. Admit to yourself that maybe it's not such a great feeling and you should try to change it. There are things that you can do.

Don't Be a Pusher

The first step is to stop pushing people away. Unseen vibrations are given off, telling people that you don't want them around. These intangible vibrations reduce your number of acquaintances, adding to your feeling of loneliness. These must stop. You have to learn to give off positive vibrations—the kind that welcome people instead of chasing them away.

Contact!

Once you start giving off new, more positive vibes, you'll want to make more friends. How can you meet people? You can start by getting involved in some kind of organization. This type of activity usually attracts people who are interested in being with others who share a common goal. Because you have RA, you may want to become involved in your local chapter of the Arthritis Foundation. There you'll meet other people with similar concerns (helping you to better cope with your illness). In addition, you may be able to find ways of helping others who have RA. This is a great way to develop friendships.

Try getting involved in a new learning activity or hobby. Take adult education courses, for example. This will help alleviate loneliness as well as boredom. Invite people to your home, but pace yourself so that you don't become exhausted. Most importantly, be receptive to the people that you meet. Try to see the good in everyone. Don't reject someone simply because there are some things that you don't like.

If you work at conquering loneliness, you'll feel much better about yourself and about your life. It will make life more enjoyable, despite your having RA. Give yourself and others a chance, and your feelings of loneliness will disappear, regardless of the limitations your condition has placed on you.

UPSET

Are there times when you feel unhappy but you're not really depressed? You might feel uncomfortable but not anxious. You may not know exactly what's bothering you, or what to do about it. On the other hand, you may know exactly what's wrong, but you just don't like it. You can do things, but you'd like things to feel differently. You may feel mixed up, confused, disturbed, agitated, or shaken up. This is typical of feeling upset. Can you get upset because of rheumatoid arthritis? Be serious, now!

When things happen to upset you, you may try to push them out of your mind so that you can adjust as slowly and as comfortably as possible. But eventually, you'll certainly want to come to grips with it.

Feeling upset is similar to experiencing other ''motivating'' emotions. They propel you to do something. So what should you do, now that you're all motivated? Try to figure out why you're upset. You *do* want to do something about it.

There's probably something in your life that is out of sorts. Things are not moving along smoothly. Something has upset the ''apple cart.''

Roseann was upset. A 34-year-old mother of three, she had just completed her latest car-pool adventure and was about to relax in front of her favorite soap opera. She had a gnawing feeling that things just weren't right, and this upset her. She knew she was upset when she found that she couldn't enjoy her program. My goodness, she had been hooked on this show for almost fifteen years! But she decided to turn off the T.V. and figure out what was upsetting her. After at least four commercials-worth of thought, she realized that it was her soap opera that was bothering her! She felt that the characters on the program, despite all of their script problems, were better off than she was. None of them needed medication—only she did! None of them needed daily exercises to keep their joints limber. But she did! As she thought about it, however, she realized that perhaps she was making something out of nothing. Actors and actresses have their own problems. So what if she also had something she must learn to live with? Medication and exercise were keeping her condition in check. She might not like it, but she needed it. She quickly noticed that she was feeling much better. In fact, she was able to turn on the television and breathlessly catch the last few minutes of her show!

Once you explore your upset feeling, you can act on this in much the same way as you do in attempting to resolve other emotional concerns. If you can identify the source of your upset, then plan a strategy. Otherwise, recognize that you can't, and move on.

PART III.
Changes In General Lifestyle

14

Coping With Changes In General Lifestyle— An Introduction

So you have to make changes in some aspects of your lifestyle because of RA? Yes, that is all part of the "package." Every time you experience pain when you move, you'll be reminded of how much you have changed. However, changes may occur in anyone's life for a number of reasons. If you got a new job, you might have to wake up at a different time, go to work in a new direction by a new form of transportation, or "survive" on a higher salary. If your new job required you to move, you would have to meet a whole new group of people. If you got a new car, you'd have to get used to its new gadgets, as well as new quirks.

In your case, RA is a new addition to your life! Although it may be hard for you to try to lead a normal life when you know your condition may never be totally cured, you're not (or shouldn't be) aiming for perfection. You just want to feel better, enjoy life, and do what you can. That's reasonable, *and* achievable.

Why are lifestyle changes so important as part of the treatment program for RA? One of the main goals of management of RA is relief from, or reduction of, pain. Your lifestyle needs to be changed in order to change, reduce, or eliminate those activities that may cause you more pain. Changes in lifestyle can also help to conserve your joints, reducing the chances of developing deformities.

Because rheumatoid arthritis can affect work, family life, sexuality, social activities with friends, finances, and other aspects of day-to-day living, it's important for you to learn how to cope with changes in lifestyle. In some cases, these changes may be minimal. But you might as well understand what you can do to cope with any changes that do occur.

Your lifestyle is of your own choosing. You'll automatically take many different factors into consideration when determining what your lifestyle is and what you want it to be. You can decide how full you want your days to be. You may also decide to put things off until you "feel better." But in the case of rheumatoid arthritis, why wait? Why not try to see what you can do right now to improve the quality of your life, even while you're learning to live with RA?

MAKING SOME CHANGES

A good way to change your lifestyle is to look for ways that you can make things easier for yourself. This may allow you to continue doing much of what you want to do, without putting as much pressure on your body. In fact, as you make changes (at your own pace), you'll feel even better because you'll probably experience less discomfort. You'll make changes in lifestyle which can help you to reduce or avoid discomfort, save your energy, and protect your joints.

For people who have problems with joints, everyday activities can put stress and pressure on them. Can these activities be eliminated? Of course not. So the best approach to improving your lifestyle is to find easier ways of doing them.

For example, try to spread out your most taxing activities. Why is it necessary to do all the house cleaning in one day? Spread it out. Pace yourself. Make sure you include rest periods during the course of the day to give your joints a chance to relax. (More about this later.)

Climate Concerns

Should you move to a different climate? Are certain climates better for those with rheumatoid arthritis? For years people have believed that moving to a warm, dry climate can be helpful for RA. It is true that people who retire to such climates, or spend months at a health spa there, may feel better. However, neither the spa nor the climate has a significant effect on the course of the disease, although either may be helpful in relieving symptoms. There is no evidence that any specific kind of climate improves or cures rheumatoid arthritis.

Sure, some people may like the idea of moving. It may give them a psychological lift. In some cases, people may feel better by moving to other climates. But then again, this is true for people who *don't* have RA, as well!

In order to decide if such a move should occur, you must consider the emotional and financial factors of such a change. You'll have to change jobs, find a new place to live, and possibly even adapt a new lifestyle. You'll be leaving old family and friends behind (of course, this may be a blessing in disguise if you're leaving behind people who deserve to be left behind!).

You have to weigh the advantages of moving (such as the possibility of feeling more comfortable) and the disadvantages (such as disrupting your family). If you really are contemplating a geographical change, it's probably a good idea to take an extended vacation in that location before actually committing yourself to such a move. If a move is going to help you to feel better, you'll probably notice this during your extended vacation. But remember: On a vacation, you don't have to cook, clean, or participate in many of the other joyful chores of life. You may feel better because of less stress and less wear and tear. However, once you move, you'll have a home to fix up, a family to care for, among other responsibilities, and stress may recur.

GETTING USED TO THE CHANGES

What are some of the factors which will determine how well you'll adapt to changes in your lifestyle? There are many. For example, what were you doing before you started experiencing RA discomfort? How satisfied were you with your major vocational (job) and avocational (leisure or recreation) activities? How much education did you have? How supportive were the people close to you—both family and friends? How has your condition affected you, both physically and emotionally? These and other questions play a role in determining how you'll adjust to RA, its treatment, and the changes it necessitates. But that doesn't mean your hands are tied. You can improve the way you deal with virtually any factor.

Yes, there will be some major changes in your lifestyle. But why assume that all of them have to be negative? Isn't it possible that some of them might be for the better? Maybe you were such a hard worker that you never spent enough time with your family. If you have to cut back on your work schedule because of RA, perhaps you'll enjoy the increased time you'll have to spend with your family. Learning to take better care of yourself will pay off in the long run. So don't convince yourself that your life is ruined just because your joints are giving you a hard time! Always look at the positive in any situation.

We'll be discussing how to deal with as many of the negatives as possible.

Your head may be spinning, fearing changes that may have to take place in your activity schedule, job, or social relationships, as well as apprehension in dealing with physical discomfort, body changes, and medication—to name only a few. In fact, you may even be concerned that you won't be able to perform your normal chores and responsibilities. This concern is not unusual. Most people with RA do feel this way. But feelings improve. Being aware that you can do more also helps.

How About Denial?

What happens if you decide not to comply with necessary changes in lifestyle? This may indicate that you're trying to "deny" your problem. Denial is a very common coping strategy. But believe it or not, denial can be a positive technique. How? It can be helpful by keeping you from dwelling on problems that aren't helped by dwelling! But denial has its negative side, too. What if denial keeps you from doing what you need to do? For example, what if you don't get enough rest, or you're too active, or you don't take all your medication, or, or, or. . . . ?! This is *destructive denial*, and it can hurt you. Hopefully, the fact that you're reading this book in the first place shows that you're not really denying inappropriately. But continue to stay on top of this.

TIPS FOR CHANGE

Here are some general tips for living with RA that make sense if you need to modify your lifestyle:

- Try to plan activities in advance. Make sure that active participation is limited. Avoid excessive physical and emotional fatigue and strain.

- Reorganize rooms, work areas, and other parts of your home (and life) to maximize efficiency and convenience.

- Try to arrange your tasks so that they flow naturally and easily from one to the other. For example, try to avoid trips back and forth to different rooms of the house.

- Try to avoid carrying. When shopping, make use of shopping carts, or use bags to carry items rather than holding them in your hands.

- Try to avoid excessive bending, straining, or reaching. Sit if you can, rather than stand.

- Use support devices when appropriate in order to save unnecessary work or activity.

- Always alternate rest periods with prolonged periods of activity. For example, you might want to plan on ten minutes of rest for each hour of activity.

Coping with changes in lifestyle forms a very important part of the process we call rehabilitation. What is your goal? To help you to live as normal a life as possible despite your condition.

The remainder of this book will address many of your concerns about lifestyle changes. The remaining chapter of Part III will be concerned primarily with changes in the things you do, the way your body feels, and the way RA affects you. So read on, and let's get your act together!

15

Medication

Believe it or not, some people welcome drugs as a powerful way to control problems in the body. Others are afraid of their power, and of eventually becoming dependent on them. Still others resent the presence of any artificial substances in their bodies. Where do your feelings fit in? Regardless of what your attitudes are toward using medication, your physician has probably made it perfectly clear that you don't have much choice in the matter. One of the most important components of a comprehensive treatment program for RA is taking medication. This can be a very important part of helping you to live a more comfortable life. However, you must take your medication properly. Otherwise, it can be very dangerous.

WHAT TO TAKE?

How is it determined which medication is going to be used? Physicians need to be aware of the severity of your RA, the amount of pain you're experiencing, what other drugs you're taking, how well you take what you're supposed to take, your age and your overall health, among other factors. But even when all these factors are taken into consideration, doctors are still not sure exactly how certain medication is going to affect you. So in many cases, trial-and-error is necessary in order to determine the proper dose. You may need to try different kinds of medication over long periods of time in order to arrive at the combination that can best help your condition. This may be very frustrating, but the results are worthwhile. Make sure you understand exactly why you're taking any medication and what it's supposed to do.

HOW AND WHEN TO TAKE

Besides knowing *what* medication you're taking and *why* you're taking it, you should completely understand *when* to take it and *how*. For example, certain medication should be taken after meals. Others may be taken during a meal. Still others may have to be taken on an empty stomach. Some medication should be taken with water, some with food, and some in other ways.

So far, you know the "what" (which medication you are taking), "why" you are taking it, "when" to take it, and "how." But you also need to know "how much" to take and "how often" to take it. (It seems like "where" to take your medication is really the only thing that's left up to you!) The "how much" and "how often," of course, will be supplied by your physician, but you'll still want to understand why. Each person has different needs as far as dose and frequency are concerned. What somebody else takes, even if this person seems to have the same problem, may not necessarily be appropriate for you. The dose and the frequency of the medication can also be based on the reaction you have to it, how well it's doing what it's supposed to do, and the severity of the problem that is being treated.

Once you begin taking medication in certain dosages, don't attempt to change these doses on your own. While some medication may only be necessary for a short time, you may need other medication for life. Whatever the duration, recognize that your medication is being prescribed specifically to help you live as healthy a life as possible. Because of the chemical natures of these drugs and the way they may interact with your body, it's extremely important for you to follow your doctor's orders in taking the drugs prescribed for you. Don't mix drugs without knowing if the combination is safe. Because you may need to take many different pills, it's important that you not play with your dosage, or play with the times you take them, or move around the number of pills you take at a particular time. Follow your doctor's prescription as carefully as possible.

You probably want to take as little medication as possible. Very few physicians will keep you on high doses of any medication unless they feel it's absolutely essential. If you're taking a substantial dose of any drug, then there must be a reason for it. Don't be afraid to ask your doctor about it. Every good doctor should be able and willing to explain prescribed medication and why you need it.

SIDE EFFECTS

Most people with RA require medication, often for months or years. But that doesn't mean you're thrilled with the idea. Not too many people are. What might bother you? Well, you're probably concerned about what the medication may be doing to your body, or what the side effects may be. This is probably one of the biggest problems concerning medication. Side effects are the "less than pleasant" consequences. They indicate that a drug is interacting with your body in a way other than the way it was intended. Because medication causes chemical changes within the body, side effects may occur whenever medication is taken. Unfortunately, the more powerful the drug, the more potent the side effects. However, remember that the benefits for your body are usually much more important than any potential side effects. Otherwise, your doctor wouldn't prescribe the medication. Physicians are aware of possible side effects, and they won't prescribe any medication that's not necessary (or at higher dosages than are necessary). If side effects do have a particularly harsh impact on you, then your physician may have to weigh the advantages against the disadvantages. Be aware, however. The "side effects" of *not* following prescribed treatment may include pain, stiffness, infection, or joint damage, among other problems.

Minimizing side effects is one reason why it's important to take medication exactly the way it's been prescribed for you. Also, you should report any medication difficulties you experience to your physician. (More about specific side effects later in this chapter.)

GETTING DOWN TO SPECIFICS

Let's talk about some of the medication for RA. The goal? You want to cope with any medicine you have to take as part of your life.

RA DRUGS ARE FOR INFLAMMATION AND PAIN

Let's review our earlier discussion of inflammation. Inflammation is usually part of the normal healing process. If tissues are wounded or bacteria invades the body, the body increases blood flow to that area. Inflammatory cells are mobilized to help repair the affected areas. Inflammation causes that particular area to become tender, warm, red, and often swollen.

In RA, inflammation causes damage. Inflammation is also a frequent cause of the pain that is experienced in RA. This inflammation can occur in either the joints, the surrounding tissues, or both. So an important goal of treatment is to suppress this inflammation and reduce pain. In addition, if pain is relieved, the stiffness and swelling that may accompany inflammation have a better chance of improving.

Some of the medication that has been helpful in treating RA can be divided into six categories:

•Aspirin

•Non-steroidal anti-inflammatory drugs (NSAIDS)

•Disease-slowing/remission-inducing drugs

•Corticosteroids

•Immunosuppressants

•Analgesics (for pain)

Aspirin

Aspirin is part of the family of salicylates, and is considered the most important drug in the world. That's a pretty bold statement (but true!). Although it's considered a safe and effective drug, it is a powerhouse. Aspirin often begins drug therapy for rheumatoid arthritis. Furthermore, it's estimated that about half of all those who suffer from RA will be helped by aspirin alone.

Virtually every American family has aspirin in its medicine chest at home. However, if aspirin is going to be used as part of treatment for rheumatoid arthritis, it should not be on a self-prescribed basis. It can be very harmful, and has to be taken carefully. Any medication used for treatment should be done only by a doctor's prescription and under his supervision.

How Does It Work?

How does aspirin "know" if it will simply be an analgesic to control pain, or whether it can also act as an anti-inflammatory? The difference is in the dosage! At low dosages, aspirin can help to reduce pain. How? It acts on the central nervous system and reduces your ability to feel pain. But if aspirin is going to be effective in reducing inflammation, a higher dose is needed. Why? Higher levels of aspirin are necessary to block the production of prostaglandins. These are the chemicals that help trigger and prolong the inflammatory process.

Prostaglandins are substances which are released wherever you experience inflammation. These prostaglandins seem to increase the pain you experience because they sensitize nerve endings. As aspirin interferes with the production of prostaglandins, it also blocks pain and reduces inflammation.

Dosage?

The correct dosage of aspirin is the one that you can best tolerate. In other words, you should try to keep the dosage of aspirin just below the level at which unpleasant side effects (such as nausea or ringing in the ears) occur.

After taking two tablets of aspirin (10 grains), you've usually reached the limit in pain-killing ability. If you take more aspirin, you probably won't get much more pain relief. You can usually take aspirin every four hours. Why? Because it tends to "wear off" in that time.

However, if you're going to use aspirin as an anti-inflammatory, you may need a daily dose of anywhere from 10 to 20 of the five-grain tablets in order for it to have an impact on your inflammation. You must continue to take this amount every day for weeks if you're going to maximize its effectiveness. Aspirin levels in the body must accumulate and remain high for a period of time before the drug is at its most effective level in treating inflammation. When the aspirin is finally at this level, it must remain there even if you feel better. If you stop taking aspirin or reduce your dosage, the body levels of aspirin will decrease, prostaglandins may increase, and symptoms may return.

Fortunately, aspirin is not an addictive drug. Nor does it seem to lose its effectiveness over time. Although some people find that taking a particular medication often enough leads to a need for more of it to do the same job, it doesn't seem to work that way with aspirin.

Should you take generic aspirin? Most physicians feel that there is nothing wrong with this. As a matter of fact, they may advise you to do so because you will save on costs and still get the same quality. But if you were doing well on a brand name aspirin and you then began to flare up when you switched to a generic aspirin, it could be that the generic brand had less strength or effectiveness.

Side Effects

There are possible side effects to taking aspirin. Unfortunately, stomach upset is a common side effect of aspirin. You may also experience nausea or indigestion. Vomiting may occur. Usually, taking aspirin with food, milk or an antacid may alleviate some of these side effects. Sometimes it can be avoided by using special types of coated aspirin. Liquid aspirin or time-release aspirin may also help to avoid an upset stomach, as may buffered aspirin or aspirin mixed with antacids.

Another side effect from high doses of aspirin is tinnitus, a ringing or buzzing in the ears. Dizziness, slight loss of hearing, or slight changes in vision may also result from high levels of aspirin. Aspirin can also cause a low grade loss of blood from the stomach. While not indicating that an ulcer is present, these surface "burns" from aspirin can lead to a low red blood count (anemia). Black stool may be a sign of blood loss. Sometimes, lightheadedness, increased fatigue, and pallor may indicate that anemia is present. However, if aspirin dosage is lowered or stopped, these side effects practically always go away. But please tell your doctor if any of these symptoms occur.

Any Problems?

There are some people who should not take aspirin. Asthma sufferers may not be able to tolerate it. Aspirin may cause serious bleeding and possibly even hemorrhaging. People with gastrointestinal problems should use it only with great caution. People who are taking other types of medication, such as blood thinners, may also be advised to avoid aspirin.

People who are allergic to aspirin (although this does not occur very often) must avoid it. There is a difference between side effects and allergies. This knowledge can mean the difference between eliminating a drug as part of your treatment program and simply adjusting the dosage or using other manipulations to enable you to use the medication. Symptoms that indicate an allergic reaction include a rash, a runny nose, or wheezing. On the other hand, symptoms such as ringing in the ears, headache, nausea, abdominal pain, or stomach upset are simply side effects.

Why is this especially important to remember? Because of the high dosages of aspirin necessary for treating RA, many people will develop some side effects. If this occurs, talk to your doctor. You may be advised to reduce your dosage slightly in order to determine exactly what the best dosage is for you.

Don't give up on aspirin too quickly. Different brands may reduce the side effects. However, if you experience any of the allergic symptoms mentioned above, these can be more serious. You should then stop taking aspirin and notify your physician immediately.

What About Tylenol?

Medication such as Tylenol (acetoaminophen), which is a pain reliever that doesn't contain aspirin, can reduce pain but will have no
effect on inflammation. As a result, it's probably not really as effective as aspirin in treating RA.

Non-Steroidal Anti-Inflammatory Drugs (NSAIDs)

Non-steroidal anti-inflammatory drugs (NSAIDs) are used to reduce
the inflammation and pain common in RA. NSAIDs were cleverly
named because they reduce inflammation, but don't contain steroids!
They also work in different ways.

Comparing Aspirin and NSAIDs

Aspirin is actually a type of NSAID. However, it's usually considered
separately from the other drugs in this category. How are aspirin and
NSAIDs similar? In general, NSAIDs have comparable effects to aspirin in reducing pain and inflammation. They also work in the same
way—by blocking the formation of prostaglandins.

However, there are some important differences between aspirin
and NSAIDs. Aspirin can be obtained over the counter. On the other
hand, most NSAIDs require a doctor's prescription. They usually cost
more than aspirin, too. But NSAIDs may be easier to take since you
don't have to swallow as many tablets—or as often.

Examples of NSAIDs

There are many different types of NSAIDs. The main difference is in
their chemical molecular structure. (Sorry, further information on
this point is slightly beyond the scope of this book!)

Some of the more common NSAIDs are listed below alphabetically.
The names given first are the brand names, followed by the generic
names in parentheses. Newer NSAIDs are coming out all the time.

• Butazolidin (phenylbutazone)

• Clinoril (sulindac)

• Dolobid (diflunisal)

• Feldene (piroxicam)

•Indocin (indomethacin)

•Meclomen (meclofenamate)

•Motrin, Rufen (ibuprofen)

•Nalfon (fenoprofen)

•Naprosyn (naproxen)

•Orudis (ketoprofen)

•Tandearil (oxyphenbutazone)

•Tolectin (tolmetin)

Any Problems?

As with aspirin or any of the other medication discussed, NSAIDs do have side effects. Some of the more common ones are stomach pains and cramps, nausea, vomiting, diarrhea, constipation, bleeding from the stomach, and ulcers. Headaches, ringing in the ears, and blurred vision may also occur. And, as in certain people who develop aspirin allergies, allergic-like symptoms can develop. If this occurs, the medication should be stopped and a physician notified immediately.

Disease-Slowing/Remission-Inducing Drugs

The drugs in this category do more than just relieve pain and reduce inflammation. They also attempt to modify or slow down the progression of the disease. This category includes anti-malarial drugs, gold, and penicillamine.

These drugs are used most often in trying to control RA when other drugs such as NSAIDs have not been successful. Doctors believe that these drugs may slow down the progression of the disease, although it's still not completely understood how this occurs.

These next two categories of drugs are used when conservative therapy is not doing the proper job in treating RA. More drastic measures of treatment can no longer be postponed. What leads to this conclusion? For one thing, the disease may be progressing. It may seem to be out of control. It may be harder for you to move. There may be more pain, stiffness, or damage in your joints. Additional joints may be affected. Organs may be involved. Fatigue may increase and there may be longer, more consistent low-grade fevers.

Any Problems?

All the drugs in this category have to be taken for several months—often as long as eight months or more—before they really do their job. Why? Because it takes a long time for them to accumulate in the bloodstream. Ironically, for this reason their good effects and side effects may be noticed for a long period of time even *after* you've stopped taking them.

Anti-Malarials

The primary anti-malarial drug used is Plaquenil. The generic name for Plaquenil is hydroxychloroquine. Originally, these drugs were developed to treat malaria. Almost accidentally, it was found that they could occasionally reduce the symptoms and slow the progression of RA.

Most people can tolerate Plaquenil pills. However, there are some possible side effects, such as an upset stomach or skin rashes. The most serious side effect of Plaquenil is gradual damage to the retina of the eye, possibly leading to loss of vision in extreme cases. This side effect, fortunately, is very uncommon. Therefore, if you're taking anti-malarials, you need to have regular eye examinations.

Gold and Penicillamine

Gold salts and penicillamine are two different kinds of drugs. However, because they have so many similarities (both good and bad), we'll talk first about the factors they share in common.

Both gold salts and penicillamine can actually lead to remission. However, you may have to maintain the drugs in order to continue the remission. Both gold therapy and penicillamine can take a number of months before reaching therapeutic levels. These drugs can be very effective in reducing inflammation. They may be able to slow down the joint destruction process which often occurs in RA.

The first step in determining whether or not these drugs work is to see if you can tolerate them. Approximately 25% of those people who try them will not be able to continue using them because of side effects.

Happily, in some cases, if you have a bad reaction to one you may still be able to tolerate the other. Or if one doesn't work well, the other may. Which should be tried first, gold salts or penicillamine? There is no clear-cut answer. In England, penicillamine is frequently used first. In the United States, gold is frequently used first!

Gold Therapy

Gold is injected into the muscles and requires weekly visits to your doctor until, after a while, the frequency of visits can be reduced. It may be costlier than penicillamine because of the expenses of necessary blood tests.

Gold salts are also available in capsule form—Ridura (auranofin). Usually, by taking it twice per day, improvement can begin in about 12 to 16 weeks. Some side effects seem to be less common than with injectable gold. However, diarrhea is more common.

In some cases, gold therapy (also called chrysotherapy) can be very helpful for treatment of rheumatoid arthritis and even JRA. Interestingly, gold has *not* been found to be effective for most other forms of arthritis.

It still isn't understood how gold therapy works. Research has shown that gold injections can help some people with RA who have not been helped by other medication. However, this treatment usually isn't used until it's been proven that other medication doesn't work.

When gold therapy is successful, rheumatoid arthritis symptoms can gradually decrease. But relief comes very slowly if it's going to come at all. This can be very frustrating. Because gold accumulates slowly in the body, it is rare for positive effects to be seen within the first 10 weeks or so of treatment. Thereafter, improvement may continue slowly.

Gold is usually given along with aspirin, NSAID's or corticosteroids. Such medication is often used at the same time as the gold treatment, especially because it takes so long for gold to work effectively. If the gold does eventually work, then the other medication may be eliminated.

How Does Gold Treatment Begin?

If your physician is determined to try gold injections, a number of factors must be taken into consideration. These include how many joints are affected, which joints are affected, how severe your symptoms are, your overall state of health, and what your joints look like when x-rayed.

Gold is usually started at a low dose and increased over two or three weeks to reach the steady injection level. If there are no problems, injections are given weekly for anywhere from 15 to 30 weeks. If there are signs of improvement, injections may then be reduced to every two weeks, every three weeks, and eventually, every four weeks. It may be continued for a long period of time (years!), depending on your needs. If gold treatment is effective for you, you'll probably stay on it as long as it works (unless side effects occur that require it to be stopped).

What Are The Side Effects?

The major side effects of gold include skin problems (such as rashes), effects on your kidneys (nephritis is a condition leading to protein spilling into the urine), and problems with bone marrow affecting your blood cells. Blood cell problems are the most dangerous. Either white blood cells or platelets may be affected. The bone marrow may stop making that particular blood cell. If the white blood cells are not made, your body becomes more vulnerable to infection. This can become serious and, in some cases, even fatal. If platelets are not made, your body loses the ability to control clotting. As a result, serious bleeding can occur. This can also be fatal. On rare occasions, liver or lung damage may occur. Fortunately, these problems usually reverse themselves when the drug is stopped. However, this reversal may take a period of time during which you are "at risk."

The skin rash that may result from gold salts is usually itchy with big, red, scaly blotches. If the rash remains mild, gold salt injections may continue, especially if they're working. However, serious rashes may require a discontinuation of treatment.

Because many of the side effects occur in the initial phases of treatment, doctors can usually tell fairly quickly whether or not gold salts can be tolerated, or if they have to be discontinued.

If you are on gold therapy, you'll need regular laboratory tests to check for blood or kidney side effects at an early stage.

Penicillamine

Penicillamine can relieve joint pain, swelling, and stiffness, but usually only after several months. Unfortunately, it doesn't help everybody. Like other drugs in this category, side effects may require you to stop taking it.

Penicillamine is available in tablet (Depen) or capsule (Cuprimine) form. Penicillamine dosage is usually built up gradually over a period of months to a point where some patients are taking either three or four pills (750 mg to 1,000 mg) per day. If remission does occur, this dosage (or a lower one) can be continued for an indefinite period of time.

Although penicillamine is a distant cousin to penicillin, it isn't the same kind of drug. You can still take penicillamine if you are allergic to penicillin.

The side effects of penicillamine are very similar to those of gold injections. The most common ones are skin rash, kidney problems, and a decreased production of blood cells. Like gold, penicillamine may damage bone marrow. Fever, rashes, chills, sores in the mouth, stomach upset, sore throat, loss of taste, muscle weakness, easy bruising, and bleeding are other possible side effects. There may be problems with connective tissue if penicillamine is used. As a result, a cut will heal more slowly and a scar may not have the same strength as it would if you were not taking penicillamine. So if you ever need stitches and you're on penicillamine, it may be a good idea to keep them in for a longer period of time. Expect a wound to heal more slowly. Because there are so many possible (and dangerous) side effects, a physician's supervision is essential.

Corticosteroids

Corticosteroids (called steroids, for short) have been shown to be effective in treating rheumatoid arthritis. However, they must be taken carefully because there can be severe side effects. This is unfortunate because corticosteroids are the most effective anti-inflammatory drugs known. Although they can relieve symptoms very effectively, they do not stop the underlying cause of the disease.

Corticosteroids are hormones that were originally discovered to be produced by the cortex of the adrenal glands. Nowadays all corticosteroids used in the treatment of disease are produced synthetically.

Steroids are very strong drugs. They can quickly reduce pain and inflammation, allergic reactions, asthma attacks, and colitis attacks. There are occasions when steroids are used for short periods of time if an individual is experiencing a severe flare-up of symptoms.

The big problem with steroids lies in the serious group of side effects that may occur, especially if they are used for a long period of time. As a result, steroids are primarily used when other medication doesn't work, or if the RA is severe (especially where vital organs are involved).

Dosage

What dose of steroids should you take? Your physician will consider many factors including the severity of your condition, your weight, habits, and age (among other things).

How Are Steroids Taken?

There are three ways that steroids may be taken. First, you can take them by mouth. Because they can make your stomach feel like the inside of Mount St. Helens, taking steroids with food can help. The steroid that is most often given by mouth is prednisone or prednisolone, although there are other forms including dexamethasone, hydrocortisone, triamcinolone, and betamethasone (that's a mouthful, isn't it???).

Second, steroids may be injected into a muscle (your arm or buttock, for example). The medicine then spreads through the body to help suppress inflammation wherever it occurs.

Third, you may receive injections into the inflamed area. Occasionally in RA, local injections of steroids into the affected joint can be helpful. This can be better than taking steroids by mouth because side effects can be reduced. Injections can relieve symptoms very effectively, but usually only for a short period of time.

There are a few problems with steroid injections, though. The primary problem is the possibility of joint infection where the needle enters the body. Another problem is that repeated injections may cause cartilage damage or destruction. Finally, if a number of joints are affected by RA, it may be unwise or even impossible to inject each joint.

Another way to "administer steroids" is to receive an injection of ACTH (adrenal cortical stimulating hormone). This is given to try to stimulate your own adrenal glands to increase their own natural production of hormones. Unfortunately, ACTH isn't considered a highly effective method for stimulating steroid production.

There is quite a bit of controversy as to whether or not steroids should be used in RA. Some people feel that they should almost never be used. Others feel that they should be used only if nothing else works, and then only in small doses. Still others feel that steroids could be used in low doses when you start taking slow-acting medication like gold, or that steroids should be reserved for short-term use only during flare-ups.

Side Effects

Taking steroids is not all "peaches and cream!" As with any medication, side effects can be a problem. The potential side effects vary from person to person. You may find your abdomen or your cheeks swelling. This is the "moon-face" syndrome, common in individuals taking high dosages of steroids for long periods of time. Not everyone using steroids experiences this swelling. Some don't experience it at all. Others may experience very noticeable changes even with small dosages. Can you imagine how depressing this can be, especially if you're sensitive about your looks or weight? Other side effects may include changes in hair growth (slow growth, loss of hair, or more hair growing on your face and body), an effect on injuries (slower healing, easier bruising), high blood pressure, a weakening of the bones (osteoporosis), cataracts, increased chance of infection, depression, and in some uncommon cases, stomach bleeding (among others).

Another problem is that steroids may mask symptoms—ones which may indicate the presence of other chronic or acute conditions. Extensive use of steroids have, on occasion, led to cases of diabetes mellitus, and may cause ulcers or aggravate already-existing ones. Your blood pressure may rise from steroid use, so keep monitoring it. Occasionally, emotional problems or other highly individual reactions may occur.

Nobody develops all these side effects, and usually they will only occur if you have used steroids for a long period of time. Unfortunately, not too much can be done about these side effects. You'll have to bear with them until steroid dosages can safely be reduced. This takes time.

The side effects of steroids have taught us an important lesson. It may not be a good idea to get too excited about any new medication that comes on the market for the treatment of RA. When steroids were first introduced as a treatment for RA, everyone became very excited because symptoms disappeared quickly. However, after a period of time, side effects became more obvious. As more time went by, the seriousness of these side effects became evident. So if you use a new drug—one that has not been available for a long period of time—there are no long-term studies to indicate what the side effects are going to be like.

Immunosuppressants

Immunosuppressants (also called cytotoxic or anti-cancer drugs) are very powerful, but also far from ideal. They are extremely potent, have considerable risks of unpleasant side effects and, in some cases, can be dangerous. Many physicians believe that they are too powerful to be used for RA. The drugs in this group are often used in individuals who receive organ transplants to prevent rejection of the donor organ. They have been used for many years to treat many different cancers. They have recently been found effective for people who have RA, lupus, and other severe autoimmune conditions. Because they are so powerful and potentially dangerous, they are usually used only if other milder drugs are not effective or if the disease appears to be aggressive. The most commonly-used immunosuppressant for RA is Imuran (azathioprine), although other drugs in this group are Cytoxan (Cyclophosphamide), Methotrexate, or Chlorambucil.

What Do They Do?

Immunosuppressants are used to reduce the effectiveness of the body's immune system. Under normal conditions, your immune system keeps bacteria, viruses and other germs from taking over. In RA, the drugs stop the cell action which is involved in the inflammation. You might receive dosages of these drugs to fight the rebelling white blood cells which may be causing your joint damage. The big problem with these drugs is that, since the immune system is being suppressed, it is less able to fight off infection or protect your body from other possible problems. Because of this, immunosuppressive drugs are usually only used in severe or life-threatening cases.

Problems?

So what are the side effects of immunosuppressants? There may be a decreased bone marrow production of cells. As a result, there could be a drop in the platelet, red blood cell, or white blood cell count. This can significantly lower your body's ability to resist infection. Physicians certainly don't want to make you even more vulnerable! Other side effects include vomiting, nausea, diarrhea, and heartburn. Skin rashes, easy bruising and bleeding, hair loss, blood in the urine or stool, damage to lungs, kidneys, liver, and ulcers can also be a problem. Finally, there may be a slightly increased chance of developing cancer by using immunosuppressive drugs.

In addition, these drugs have been known to interact dangerously with many other drugs. So physicians are very careful in monitoring them. (But at least they don't cause diabetes, cataracts, weight gain, and all those other steroid side effects.)

Analgesics (Painkiller Drugs)

Painkillers are usually a less significant part of RA treatment programs. Why? There are four main disadvantages to the use of painkillers. First, they don't do anything for the RA at all. They simply cover it up. Second, the importance of pain is that it tells you that there is something wrong with your body. Painkillers hide this information. If you cover up the pain, you may be doing additional damage to your body without being aware of it. A third problem with painkillers is that you become used to them fairly quickly. As a result, after a long period of time they are not nearly as effective. You need more of them to produce the same effect. This is known as "tolerance." You may need to continuously increase your dose so that it keeps working, and this leads to the possibility of addiction. This may be psychological as well as physiological! The fourth problem is that painkillers can have significant side effects, including upset stomach, constipation, or mental changes. Most of the side effects merely add to the problems that come with your condition.

One of the best-known examples of painkillers is the acetaminophen family, better known as Tylenol or Datril. They may be useful in treating RA, but are better suited for other arthritic conditions. Other analgesics include propoxyphene (better known as Darvon or Darvocet), codeine, oxycodone (better known as Percodan or Percocet), Demerol, and Talwin.

Additional Medication 'Minders

Once you've begun a medication program, make sure you let your physician know how effective the drugs are in helping you with your condition. Any significant changes in your health, whether good or bad, should be reported to your physician. In this way, your doctor will be best able to decide whether or not to keep prescribing the medication you're taking.

You may find that dealing with the same drugstore and pharmacist is very comforting. The more time you spend there, the better the pharmacist will get to know you and your specific case. You'll have somebody else looking out for your welfare in addition to your physician!

It is almost impossible for any physician to keep up with all the thousands of different types of prescription drugs on the market. However, this is the pharmacist's specialty. Frequently, pharmacists know even more than physicians as far as what drugs can go together and what drugs interact dangerously. So it can be very helpful for you to develop a good working relationship with your local pharmacist. Not only will your pharmacist be able to tell you about the medication that has been prescribed for you, but he may be able to help you reduce costs. Occasionally, generic products may be available which cost less than brand-name products. However, in some individuals the generic drug will not work as well as the brand-name medication. If you have a good relationship with your pharmacist, you will find it a lot easier to get the medication you need.

What happens if you go into a pharmacy with a prescription and the pharmacist wants to substitute another drug (or a generic one) for the medication that was originally prescribed for you? There may be nothing wrong with this, but it would probably be a good idea to consult your physician before making such a substitution.

You may experience certain emotional reactions to taking medication (such as depression or anger). This must be dealt with. (If necessary, look back at the chapters on coping with your emotions.) Remember: If it's really necessary for you to take medication, you might as well let it do what it's supposed to. Accept it and don't let it bother you.

A FINAL COMMENT

Research often produces new drugs in the fight against RA. By the time you read this book there may be additional drugs on the market that are far superior to the ones you've been taking. There is nothing wrong with discussing medication with your physician, asking if new drugs are on the market. But remember—this doesn't mean that they are necessarily good for you.

This chapter doesn't include all medication used by people with RA. Instead, it emphasizes the more common ones. But at least this information will help you to become more familiar with the ones you may hear about. So if your doctor prescribes something new, ask about it. Not only will you probably feel better physically, but you'll know why!

16

Diet

Food, glorious food! Do you like to eat? It's one of the great pleasures of life. But you might be afraid that your diet will have to change because of your RA. Or maybe friends and family members have told you that you should change the way you eat.

Is there any particular diet that is most appropriate for RA? The answer is a resounding *no*! There is no particular diet or food that will either help or hurt RA. Of course, it's important that your diet be nutritionally sound and well-balanced. A proper diet ensures that we consume all of the necessary vitamins, minerals, and supplements.

If you have RA, you may occasionally experience certain nutritional deficiencies. During a flare-up, your body may use up certain nutrients at different rates of speed than normal. This may lead to your feeling more fatigued and tired than usual. Therefore, your physician may suggest that you supplement your nutritional intake in order to make up for these deficiencies. However, this does not mean that dietary changes or supplements are going to eliminate or cure your RA! So even though RA is not caused by dietary deficiencies, you'll still want to eat a well-balanced diet as part of your complete treatment package for taking care of your RA.

There's one other main dietary note to keep in mind. You'll want to lose weight if you are overweight. Why? Added weight can put more pressure on your already affected joints. If you are overweight, don't put all the blame for this on your RA! Your weight may increase or decrease and your appetite may change, but this fluctuation may have nothing to do with your medical condition. Maybe your weight is fluctuating because of weekend binges! Maybe you've gone to some food orgies! Maybe emotional crises have caused you to overeat. So one of the most important things you can do to help stay as healthy as possible is to eat properly and keep your weight at the proper level. Don't be a junk-food junkie, because then you'll be taking a chance of hurting yourself.

Because diet is on everybody's mind these days, it becomes a very good source for quacks. Frequently, you'll hear of miracle remedies involving certain types of dietary modifications which are "destined" to cure your RA symptoms. Unfortunately, no diet has yet been invented that can do any such thing.

The types of diets that have been suggested by quacks include fish diets, vitamins, vegetarian diets, fresh fruits and laxatives, oils, low-fat, high-fat, low-protein, high-protein, and every other combination that you can imagine. But you know by now that there is no such cure for arthritis.

The moral? Eat healthy, eat in moderation, and enjoy!

17

Physical
Changes

Unfortunately, there may be some physical changes in your body because of RA. Although effective management may stop or slow down the progression of RA, it may not reverse damage which has already occurred. So physical changes can take place, and they may play a major role in the psychological adjustment to your condition.

What can you do? Well, you won't be able to do something about all the physical changes, but many of them can be helped. So first concentrate on those things you *can* do something about. Then work on learning how to accept and live with the ones you can't change. That may seem like a tall order, but what choice do you have? After all, you're still the same person inside, aren't you (and I'm not talking about your joints!)?

Let's discuss three of the more common physical changes that may occur with RA—fatigue, joint problems, and rheumatoid nodules—and how to better cope with them. If there's anything you can do about them, suggestions will be offered. If not, at least you're learning more about the changes, and you're becoming aware that you're not alone in experiencing them.

FATIGUE

Do you become more tired, more easily? Does your bed seem to be your favorite place in the whole world? If so, you're not alone. Fatigue (yawn!) is a very common problem for individuals with RA. You may find that simply getting up, washing, and getting dressed makes you tired. You may be pooped for the rest of the day. Your body simply may not be able to do what you want it to do. Fatigue

131

encompasses the loss of that "get up and go" feeling—not only tiredness or sleepiness.

Most people think of fatigue as negative. This is not always the case. It can be positive. How? Fatigue is your body's way of telling you that you need rest. If you didn't feel tired, you would push yourself too much! Then you'd certainly feel the effects. So if you feel fatigue, you should listen to your body.

What Causes It?

Usually in a situation such as RA, fatigue is caused by the disease. This is a physical kind of fatigue, and the best way to treat it is to treat the disease that is causing the fatigue. However, this may take some time.

Of course, fatigue can be caused by doing *too* much! Or it can occur even if you haven't been too active. In this case, the fatigue can be due to other factors such as disease activity, emotional factors, anemia, or medication.

Consider the possibility that your fatigue may be emotional rather than physical. In other words, you're tired because of the way you feel emotionally—not so much because of physical exhaustion. If this is the case, try to determine what emotional reactions are contributing to the fatigue. For example, fatigue could be due to depression, boredom, worry, or just unhappiness. Then you can work on improving these feelings.

What Can You Do?

What's the best way to cope with fatigue? Rest. (Clever!) A good night's sleep, or short naps during the day, are great for coping with fatigue.

Although rest may not make fatigue problems disappear, they can certainly help. If fatigue is a message saying that your body is unable to do as much as you want it to do, rest is certainly an important way to gain more control. One problem, however, is that *too much rest* can only lead to more fatigue! This can start a vicious cycle.

Fatigue can also be reduced by efficient planning and pacing. Figure out what you have to do. Schedule activities so that you're not doing too many strenuous things in a row. Make sure you intersperse rest periods with any strenuous activities you need to do. And be flexible. You can never be sure when you're going to have energy, or when you're going to feel too fatigued to do anything.

Know your priorities. Focus on the top priorities while you still have the energy. In this way, if fatigue sets in, it will be the less significant activities that need to be delayed.

Other techniques which you have learned in becoming an "efficiency expert," such as reorganizing your house and making things more convenient, will also help you to do more and feel less fatigued. Don't feel like you have to make all these changes by yourself. Getting advice from professionals can help you to improve the quality of your day-to-day functioning.

JOINT PROBLEMS

Joint problems are among the most common physical complaints in rheumatoid arthritis. Other than pain, stiffness (especially in the morning) is a very common characteristic of RA. This stiffness may last for much longer than a few minutes—possibly for two or three hours or more. Morning stiffness is sometimes called the "gel phenomenon." After awakening in the morning or after sitting or standing still for a short period of time, your body may seem to stiffen up. It may be harder to move. After a period of loosening up, movement may become easier and less painful. The synovial fluid seems to gel during a period of immobility, and movement gets it flowing smoothly once again.

What Causes These Problems?

As we've discussed earlier, joint pain, stiffness, and reduced mobility are usually caused by inflammation. But rather than repeating all the exciting effects of inflammation, let's talk about what can be done to help!

What Can You Do?

The primary treatment for joint problems involves medication and physical therapy (both discussed in other chapters). But there are other things that can be done, too.

Supportive devices such as canes, crutches, walkers, splints, or braces can help joints such as the hands, ankles, feet, hips, or knees. They preserve and protect them (sounds like the U.S. Constitution!) and allow for as much functional mobility as possible. These devices may also help by spreading out the weight that would be placed on any weightbearing joints.

What can be done about joint stiffness? Remember that one of the best ways to treat morning stiffness is to treat your RA in general. It's possible that if you haven't been taking proper care of yourself, stiffness may serve as a reminder. Try to loosen up slowly, gradually, and gently, but recognize that it may still take time for your joints to become more mobile. Make sure you're taking medication at the proper times.

A warm (not hot) bath or shower may be helpful. Gentle exercises may help to loosen you up. Anticipate that you will experience a certain amount of stiffness each day. Work it out of your joints as comfortably as you can.

If you find that morning stiffness is lasting longer and longer each day, consult your physician. It may be necessary to change certain medication or other parts of your treatment program.

Principles of Joint Protection

Regardless of what you do, you'll want to do everything you can to protect your joints from further damage or stress. Some medication may even work better if you protect an inflamed joint from excessive motion or weight bearing. So it can be very helpful to become aware of some of the basic principles of joint protection.

- Try to use the strongest or largest joint possible when you have to do something. For example, your wrist is a larger joint than your fingers. Therefore, when possible, use your wrist instead of your fingers. In the same vein, try using your shoulder instead of your elbow, and so on.

- Try to avoid placing too much pressure against small joints of the hand (such as the backs or pads of your fingers). This can put too much stress on the weakened joints of the knuckles and may result in a deformity. Use your palms instead of your fingers where at all possible.

- Try not to allow joints to remain in one particular position for too long. In other words, if you have to hold something—whether it's a cup, glass, book, or cards—try not to hold it in the same position for too long. Change positions as often as you can (within reason).

- Try to extend your joints as much as possible in all activities. People with joint problems tend to keep them slightly contracted (flexed). Why? A slight contraction of the joints is usually more comfortable if you're in pain, if the joint is inflamed, or even if a joint is normal.

This is because flexing makes use of stronger muscles than extension. Extending your joints (opening them fully) can keep joints mobile even though it may be slightly less comfortable when you do so. Interestingly enough, extended joints may require less strain.

• Avoid lifting whenever you possibly can, for it is a very stressful activity.

RHEUMATOID NODULES

The nodules, or bumps under the skin, which may develop in RA, are most commonly seen near the elbows, knees, or ankles, in the tendons of the fingers, or in the back of the head. Sometimes they can even occur in the lung. They are most common near your elbows because pressure is often placed here. They may vary from the size of a pea to that of a walnut, or even larger. These nodules can come and go during the course of your illness. They usually don't cause problems, although they may occasionally become infected, tender, and painful.

Rheumatoid nodules are caused by the inflammation of small blood vessels. Surgery is usually not advisable. However, surgery may be needed to prove that a nodule is the rheumatoid nodule and not another type of growth. Surgery for rheumatoid nodules would be primarily for cosmetic reasons, since function and mobility is usually adequate and pain is usually not a problem. Even if surgery is performed, they tend to grow back.

A PHYSICAL FINALE

So there are changes as a result of RA. This chapter has included only some of the more common ones. Some of them are preventable, some are not. Some are treatable and curable, some are not. But once again, what's the alternative? You do want to learn how to cope with RA, and the changes that result from it. That's why you're reading this book, right?

18

Activities

What to do, what to do? Sure you have RA, but what does this mean in terms of the basic activities in your life? What *can* you do and what *can't* you do? Even if you feel wonderful, you'll still want to curtail any vigorous activities. You don't want to put any strain on your joints. In fact, you may not even have the strength!

Each person is different. The kinds of things you did before beginning treatment for RA can influence what you can or want to do now. Your current physical condition is also a determining factor. For example, if you've had joint replacement surgery, you'll want to hold off on most exertions until healing has taken place and your doctor has given you the green light (or even a cautious yellow) to continue. So let's discuss some of the more important types of activities that people participate in.

WORKING

Working can be very important for you. Besides being your source of income (can't overlook that!), you do want to feel like your life is proceeding as usual. You may be concerned (an understatement!) if your RA threatens the possibility of your working. This may interfere with your financial security.

Even though you have RA, you'll probably want to do as much of what you used to as possible. Are you afraid that you'll feel like less of a person if you have to stop working? Work is important. It helps you to feel independent. It gives you a sense of self-fulfillment. It provides more financial strength than not working, of course. And it provides a social life.

Many people question whether or not they should work. The answer: If you want to, and you need to, and you can, then you should! You may have to make some modifications because you don't want to take a chance of putting too much stress on your joints. This would only increase your pain and discomfort, and could cause further damage.

Where to Work

Five basic points may help you when you are resuming an old job or taking on a new one. First of all, ask yourself if you feel comfortable doing the job. Do you feel physically and emotionally capable? Is it something you want to do? Your condition may have made you more aware of your mortality. As a result, you might decide to start doing something you really want to do! Second, if you had been working prior to experiencing your first RA flare, will your employer take you back? Or will a new employer hire you, given your present physical condition? Should you even say anything about it? (More about this in a later chapter.) A third very important point is whether your colleagues will accept you. This, of course, does not mean that they will even notice your condition. Fourth, will your condition affect your attendance at work or your punctuality? If so, will this cause any difficulties on the job? A fifth factor that may relate to your choice of employment is the amount of stress involved. Stress is certainly a factor you'll want to minimize. Can stress exacerbate your physical condition? You may decide to change jobs if you recognize that your previous job was too stressful.

Stamina Shortage

RA may cause you to experience fatigue, depression, and adjustment problems. This may affect your work productivity, especially if your treatment has not yet been very helpful. Your work rate may slow down, you may be absent more often, and your value to the company may decrease. You simply may not feel physically able to work. You may get tired easily, and feel that you just don't have the stamina necessary to complete your job satisfactorily. You may need to be off your feet more, or you may have been told not to walk up and down stairs. If your employer is aware of any of these problems, you may be afraid that your job will be in jeopardy.

What can you do? Build up your stamina slowly. Don't expect too much at once. Pacing yourself is probably the most important thing you can do. Take frequent rest breaks to "recharge your batteries." If you're not sure how much you can do, do what you can and let the experience of pain in your body be your guide. That's one reason why it's important not to use too much pain medication. It will suppress the amount of pain that you're aware of.

There's no reason to believe that, once medication and other components of your treatment program begin to help, you won't be able to continue working. On the other hand, if you just can't succeed at your old job because of its requirements, this doesn't mean that you can't succeed at another job that requires less physical exertion.

Bending the Rules?

Employers are not required by law to make any special provisions for you because you have RA. You still have to do what you're supposed to do. However, if you're an important employee, your company will probably want to retain your services. You may be able to continue working at a particular job with only a few modifications (such as changing your chair, desk, location, or a few of the activities you used to do). Changing your hours may also be helpful.

You may be uncomfortable about approaching your employer to find out if these changes can be made. It may bother you to seek special treatment on your job, but this is something you'll have to do. If you are a valued employee, these changes may be small in comparison to the problems your company would face (such as hiring a new employee to replace you).

You may find that you have difficulty with other employees if you receive special treatment. This may not be true at all, but your anticipation or apprehension of this happening may cause problems.

Changing Jobs

Don't stay at a job if it's not right for you. Consider transferring to another one or getting additional training to move into a new job. In some cases, individuals with certain job experiences and backgrounds are unable to work in jobs for which they were trained because of their new condition. For example, Lenny (a 39-year-old father of two) had been working in construction. But doctors felt he shouldn't continue this type of work because it was too strenuous for him. It put too much pressure on his joints. Lenny became very depressed. He didn't know what else he could do. He shut down emotionally, rather than face the prospect of not being able to work. He was even afraid that he didn't have the ability to go out and get new training. How do you deal with this? One way might be to check with the Office of Vocational Rehabilitation (OVR), a government-provided service. The Office of Vocational Rehabilitation can be a very important resource in helping you get back to work. You'll find office locations throughout your state. Counselors in these offices will work with you to determine exactly what your aptitude is for different jobs. OVR will then provide you with training and support to help you obtain employment in those fields. In addition, they also provide transportation, counseling, placement, and even equipment (where necessary). If you've been having difficulty getting a new job and are not sure how to proceed, calling your local Office of Vocational Rehabilitation may be an excellent way to begin. If you need help in finding jobs that are appropriate for you, you may want to check with the State Employment Services. These services are available free of charge and have specialists that can help you to find jobs that are suitable for your needs.

Is Working Your Only Option?

What are the advantages of working? Some of the benefits are satisfaction, productivity, money, and pride. But what if you can't work? Or what if you're between jobs? A paying job is not the only type of satisfying work. There are plenty of other meaningful, productive activities that can be done voluntarily. Check with non-profit organizations, hospitals, schools, senior citizen centers, and the like. They can always use some extra help. You'll feel good about yourself, too. Volunteers can also work with religious, political, or charitable organizations.

What if you just don't want to work? Some individuals with RA are happy about not being able to work. But don't use your condition as an excuse for not working. This may indicate that something else is bothering you. You may want to explore this further.

SCHOOL

Problems with going to school are similar to those with working. Attendance may decrease because there may be times when you just don't feel up to going. You may be concerned about going to school because of physical restrictions or the reduced number of activities that you can participate in. A child who requires medication for JRA may be concerned about other students' comments while in school. Teachers should be informed so that they are made aware of these potential problems.

THERAPEUTIC RECREATION

People with RA may still be able to participate in a number of different types of activity including boating, skating, golf, tennis, and dancing. Whether or not you do depends on your condition. If you try an activity without experiencing pain, swelling, or long-lasting discomfort, you're probably o.k. On the other hand, there may be times when your condition keeps you from feeling like you can do it. However, if your doctor approves, at least you know that you can try. It's up to you and your doctor to decide which activities are best for you. Certain joints may be stressed by certain activities and, as a result, those activities should be avoided.

You're probably participating in exercises that you might normally participate in to increase muscle strength and maintain range of motion in your joints. The exercises that are found in normal hobbies and other types of pleasurable activities can actually be extensions of these exercises. This is what falls under the category of therapeutic recreation. The advantage of therapeutic recreation, therefore, is that it not only includes exercise which is important for joint mobility, but provides recreation as well.

Why is it so helpful to participate in activities which you enjoy? They can help improve your ability to take care of yourself. They can help promote and maintain your participation in the normal activities of daily living, and they can certainly provide you with benefits in both the social and psychological aspects of your life.

ACTIVITIES OF DAILY LIVING

Among the things you'll do each day are the normal, routine tasks known as the activities of daily living (ADL). But there's a problem. The pain and reduced mobility of RA may limit these activities. This can be frustrating. Why? Probably because, prior to being diagnosed, you may have taken such simple tasks for granted. The way you're feeling now, however, may make you depressed and upset, rather than enthusiastic about trying to conquer the problem.

What if you can't do what you want to do? You may not want to ask for help. You may feel that it takes away some of your dignity. This can make you very uncomfortable. However, the future can be brighter! In a very short period of time, you can reorganize your lifestyle, your house, and your daily activities, in a way that can reduce your difficulties and salvage a lot of your dignity.

But first, what ADL difficulties may you have? You may have problems getting dressed or undressed. You may have difficulty with bathroom activities, such as bathing or using the toilet. There may also be problems holding a toothbrush or comb, or washing or drying various parts of your body. You may have difficulty opening doors or turning handles. You may have problems opening jars or holding objects that would require fine motor coordination. You may have difficulty eating food or preparing it. You may have difficulty moving, walking, or going up or down stairs. But don't despair. Not all people with RA experience these problems. (And if you do, doesn't it make sense to see what you can do to improve the situation?)

Modifying your lifestyle or your home is not the same as giving in to RA. However, it may be an important part of helping you to learn to live most effectively and cope most successfully with your condition.

Easing the Load

Your goal is to make daily living as easy as possible. Why? Other than protecting your joints and relieving pain, one of the most important components in your treatment program for RA is energy conservation. So you'll want to eliminate those activities which aren't necessary and simplify those which are! Conserving your energy can be very important in helping you to reduce the stress in your joints. It can also help you to avoid much of the excessive fatigue that can be a negative factor in living with RA.

In many cases, problems with daily living can be conquered without professional help. It can be very satisfying for you to develop your own solutions to these problems. This can be one of the most important ways of coping with RA. Of course, any questions you have can be bounced off physicians, physical therapists, or occupational therapists. In fact, one of the occupational therapist's main goals is in helping you to solve all problems in daily living, especially at home or those related to your occupation. This will greatly improve your overall functioning.

Start by trying to evaluate everything you do on a day-to-day basis and seeing how you can make every single thing you do easier. Realistically, you know you cannot eliminate all of the activities that you need to do around your home. However, what's wrong with finding easier ways of doing them? Is this taking the lazy way out? Of course not. You are simply recognizing that every bit of energy you save from one activity will give you more energy to do something else.

Any specific suggestions? There are lots of things you can do to help yourself with daily living. For example, you may want to reorganize your home and your habits in such a way that makes movement easier and puts things within easy reach. You can replace small handles on drawers with bigger ones. You can lubricate drawers so that they open and close more easily. You can wear clothing that is easier to get on and off. There are a number of different types of gadgets that will make life easier for you.

You'll also want to learn how to moderate your activities. Plan them out carefully and pace yourself. One thing you may find helpful is to chart out your activities, including required activities as well as social and leisure activities. This may help you to become better organized so that you can pace yourself more effectively.

Try to plan activities in advance so you can figure out exactly how you're going to do them, what equipment you're going to need, and how much time you can spend doing them in between rest periods. This will help you to reduce the amount of strain, both physically and emotionally, and will keep you from getting overtired.

Try to reduce the amount of energy you expend in performing any activities. If necessary, modify the method that you use. Try to use any assistance devices or equipment that you can to conserve energy and protect your joints. Eliminate any unnecessary activity. Rest intermittently, frequently, and whenever needed. You'll then be able to do more of what you want or need to do. And you'll accomplish it in a healthier way.

Any activities that cause you pain should be modified as much as possible. If you've already reduced a task to the bare minimum, and absolutely can't do anything more about it, put a limit on how much pain you're going to let yourself endure. In general, you may want to avoid pain which lasts longer than 15 to 20 minutes.

Support Devices

There are many different types of support and self-help devices which can help you in your daily activities. You can buy or borrow many of them from organizations, hospitals, and volunteer agencies.

Any support devices that you purchase or develop should meet certain requirements. They should be durable, lightweight, economical, pleasant to look at, versatile and, most importantly, useful!

The support devices that you may find most helpful in daily living can be divided into five categories: (1) bath and toilet aids (such as raised toilet seats, handles, bath or shower seats, and rubber mats); (2) dressing aids (such as clothing with Velcrow fasteners instead of buttons, shoes which are easier to get on, hooks and pull strings for pulling up zippers, etc.); (3) walking aids (such as canes, crutches, walkers, sticks, or other supportive devices); (4) eating aids (such as special long-handled or thick-handled utensils); and (5) household aids (such as book rests, groping tools, or jar openers).

There are many helpful tools or devices available in each category. Going into detail about these devices, however, is beyond the scope of this book. To find out more about specific devices you can use, you may want to consult the Arthritis Foundation or other sources of support. The Arthritis Foundation publishes a self-help manual that includes types of devices, purchase prices, and resources designed to help solve many of the different problems with daily living. Also, many pharmacies and surgical supply firms have booklets for you to look at before purchasing any device.

Remember that any special devices needed to make your home more "RA-suitable" are tax-deductible because of your condition. Obtain a prescription from your physician for any necessary equipment in case it's necessary when filing your income tax returns.

How do you cope with these support devices? Remember that using a cane, crutch, splint, or any other device is not "giving in" to RA. It's not a sign of weakness. These devices do not lead to "dependency" on them; rather, they allow independence! They speed up activities, permit other activities previously too difficult to do, and help permit joint rest and protection. Does it embarrass you to have to use a cane, splint, or brace? Don't let it. Tell yourself how much it's helping you. Using one of these devices to help your joints is not dissimilar to using glasses to help your eyes! What's more important—support devices and independence, or avoiding "embarrassment" and dependence?

A FINAL EXERTION

Keeping active is a very important part of coping with RA. You want to feel productive and enjoy life. You don't want to let rheumatoid arthritis confine you to your closet. So don't let it. Do what you physically can, but *do*. . . .

19

Pain

Ouch! (Just getting you ready for this chapter!) Is rheumatoid arthritis painful? Are you kidding?! Most individuals with RA believe that the pain is the hardest thing to deal with. But the good news is that treatment for RA is designed to improve your quality of life, and decrease your discomfort.

What is pain? Pain is a type of sensation picked up by nerve endings and transmitted to the brain. This message is very important. Why? Pain is a signal from your body telling you that you're having trouble in a particular part. As a result, pain can be an important diagnostic tool. It can help you to determine the nature or severity of an illness or injury. Only after these messages travel from the site of irritation to the brain do we feel pain.

Only you know the intensity of your pain. Pain suggests that you rest the injured areas of your body so that your tissues can be repaired. It also signals you to "slow down" to prevent additional damage.

In RA, pain is an important defense mechanism. It can tell you that a joint is injured or that you're using a damaged joint too much. It can also tell you that you're interfering with the natural healing process. This is one reason why doctors don't like you trying to suppress pain using medication. If you do, you may end up being too active. For example, you may try to use sore muscles and joints the way you did before. This may cause further damage.

What can you do about your discomfort? How can you cope with it? The best way to cope with pain is to get rid of it! To do this, it's first necessary to identify the cause of the pain.

CAUSES OF YOUR PAIN

Unfortunately, it's still not completely understood what causes the pain of RA. It's possible that the pain results when the nerves in the joint become irritated. Inflammation of the synovial membrane can be a major source of pain because of the pressure created. Besides the pressure, tension and spasm in muscles or fatigue can also be contributors.

Earlier in the development of RA, pain may have only been triggered by movement. Eventually, however, pain may increase to the point where it might occur during rest periods as well.

GETTING STARTED

Once you're aware of what's causing your pain, treatment can attempt to eliminate the cause. But what if you can't do anything about the underlying source of the pain? At least you can try to get some relief from it.

How do you start? First, be aware of your pain. While this may sound strange, you'll learn to recognize whether your pain is something you can (and should) handle yourself, or if it's serious enough to be discussed with your doctor. Remember: If in doubt, check it out. Inform your doctor about the pain. Together you can work out the best ways of dealing with it.

WHEN DOES PAIN OCCUR?

Many factors may contribute to your pain. You'll want to try to control any or all of these factors in order to manage it. Remember that pain can be affected by both psychological and environmental factors. Although pain may initially be physical, emotions can quickly worsen or exacerbate the pain. So pain may also result from stress, fatigue, or depression.

Stress causes you to tense your muscles. It may make it more difficult for you to relax. This can increase the degree of pain that you're experiencing. If you're fatigued, you may feel more pain because your tissues and joints aren't getting the rest they need to repair themselves. Depression may cause you to feel more pain because it's on your mind more than it would normally be.

When you're in pain, this may increase the degree to which you experience stress, fatigue, or depression. This can lead to more pain, creating a vicious cycle.

TREATMENT FOR PAIN

There are four traditional categories of therapy for pain control: chemical (using medication), surgical, physical (physical therapy), and psychological. In general, all four therapies work by interrupting the transmission of pain messages before the brain receives and interprets them.

Medical treatment for pain generally involves medication. This can effectively control a lot of problems. For example, aspirin has been proven effective in controlling minor pain. But sometimes discomfort will continue, despite the use of medication. In extreme cases, surgery may be helpful in treating the cause of the pain. But not all conditions lend themselves to surgical treatment. So it may be necessary for you to learn other techniques for dealing with pain.

Other than medicine and surgery, what are other ways of trying to obtain pain relief? Acupuncture, chiropractic, or physical therapy techniques (such as using TENS units, heat, cold, hydrotherapy, and a proper balance of rest or exercise) can be used, as well as psychological techniques such as imagery, biofeedback, yoga, hypnosis, and relaxation. Last but not least, it's very important to maintain a positive attitude.

You can learn how to employ techniques for controlling pain from physicians, physical therapists, occupational therapists, and mental health professionals (such as psychologists who may specialize in certain pain control techniques). Or you may want to read some of the many books on pain which can be found in bookstores and libraries. A good book to read is *Free Yourself From Pain* by David Breslin. Another one is *Life Without Pain* by Richard Linchitz.

Many techniques for pain control can be applied at home, although in some cases they may achieve greater success in clinics or centers.

Despite the effectiveness of the pain control techniques mentioned in this chapter, it's important to consult your physician to make sure that any or all the techniques are appropriate for *you*. Make sure that any techniques you're thinking of using are not dangerous for you, considering your condition.

Now let's go on to discuss some of these techniques.

TENS Units

TENS stands for Transcutaneous Electrical Nerve Stimulation. These devices have been gaining popularity in helping to control pain. The TENS unit is a little box about the size of a cigarette pack which contains a generator that has wire leads with electrodes at the ends of them. The unit may have anywhere from 2 to 40 electrode wire leads. A little gel is attached to the electrodes. They're then placed on your skin, on or near the area to be treated. When you turn on the unit, a low level of electricity flows into the area from the TENS unit. This stimulates the nerve fibers and blocks the transmission of pain messages to the brain. Shocking, right? Don't worry. You probably won't even feel anything, or you may just experience a mild tingling sensation.

One of the problems with TENS units is that their effectiveness seems to decrease as time goes by. The effectiveness of the TENS unit also seems to be related to your diligence, the knowledge of your teacher, and the appropriate placing of electrodes.

If you want to get a TENS unit, you usually need a prescription from your physician. You can then be taught by a nurse or physical therapist how to place the electrodes to provide you with maximum pain relief. But it's probably a good idea to rent a machine before buying one to see if it works.

Acupuncture

Many people are very curious about the field of acupuncture. This technique consists of placing special needles in specific areas of the body. To some people, acupuncture is considered an important method of controlling pain. To others, acupuncture is simply another type of quackery that people with RA should avoid.

Research indicates that acupuncture may have very little value in the long-term treatment of RA. In some cases, there may be temporary relief from pain, but acupuncture seems to do little to stop the progression of RA or to reduce the underlying inflammation—which is the main problem of RA in the first place!

If you're considering acupuncture, it is essential that you speak to your physician first. If you are comfortable with your physician, you'll trust his or her judgment as to whether or not these techniques are appropriate for you.

Chiropractic

Some people feel that chiropractic measures can be helpful in RA. Why? The joints are the main trouble sites in RA, and their manipulation may help to make things better. There is quite a bit of concern on the part of the medical establishment, however, that manipulation of problem joints actually makes things worse. In some cases, individuals with RA may find that their disease worsens following a chiropractic manipulation. Again, a consultation with your physician is imperative.

HEAT AND COLD

Both heat and cold treatments can be beneficial in the temporary relief of painful RA symptoms. However, neither has an effect on the disease itself. If you're going to use either heat or cold, be careful! You can hurt yourself if you misuse it.

Some people seem to benefit more from heat; others seem to benefit more from cold. This may vary within you as well, depending upon the stage of your disease. There may be times when they work best in combination. At other times, different joints may benefit from different approaches.

Heat

Heat can be a very beneficial way of relaxing and soothing your muscles to relieve soreness and pain. This is called thermotherapy. It's considered to be the oldest form of pain reliever or analgesic.

Heat increases the temperature in a selected area of your body. There are two good reasons for this. One: It increases blood circulation to the area. Two: It increases the metabolic rate.

If you're using heat, you should feel comfortably warmed and relaxed. Relaxing tight muscles can increase the mobility of your joint. (This is one reason why using heat before exercise can be helpful.) Usually, positive effects from heat can be felt in about 20 minutes, give or take a few minutes. However, trial and error is necessary to find out what's best for you.

Is Heat Always Helpful?

Heat may not always be appropriate, especially during acute inflammatory phases of RA. Why? If an affected joint is treated with heat, it may aggravate the symptoms in this joint. There may be increased swelling or damage. Heat may be harder to tolerate if you're very young or very old.

If heat is going to be used, care must be taken regarding the intensity and duration of its use. Too much heat for too long a period of time is not advisable. Don't feel that if a little bit of heat is good, a lot of heat can be better. This is a good way to get burned!

Ways To Apply Heat

The methods of applying heat may be divided into two categories: moist heat or dry heat. Examples of moist heat include using hot towels (or hydrocollators), hydrotherapy, or water baths. Hydrotherapy can be used for both hot and cold applications. (More about this later.) Dry heat can be applied using heating pads, lamps, or heaters. (Obviously, if you use any electrical appliances, use them carefully!)

Is there a difference between the effectiveness of moist heat and dry heat? Not very much. Both can be effective as long as the frequency, duration of treatment, and intensity are controlled.

Some ways of applying heat may be more effective for large areas of your body; others may be more effective for small areas. Let's discuss some specific heat treatment techniques.

Hydrocollators

One way to apply moist heat is by using warm, damp towels or hydrocollators. Hydrocollators may be very helpful in relieving pain and reducing inflammation. What is a hydrocollator? The hydrocollator pack is usually made up of a cotton sack which contains a gel. That's why they may also be called "gel packs." These cotton bags are heated in hot water, wrapped in terrycloth, and applied to the painful area for about 20 minutes. The silica gel, which is contained in hydrocollator packs, can retain heat for a long period of time. Or you can make your own hot compresses of towels. This involves soaking a towel in hot water, then wringing it out and applying it to the painful area.

If you use hydrocollator packs or hot compresses, be careful to avoid burns! In general, a good way to avoid burns and retain heat for longer periods of time is to use plastic sheets or dry towels wrapped around the hot compress.

Warm Baths

A warm bath in the morning is a great idea. Not only can it be very helpful in reducing the stiffness and pain you'll feel upon awakening, but you'll get clean in the bargain! Hot showers can also reduce stiffness. Many muscles can be relaxed at the same time. Usually, baths or showers should last no longer than 20 minutes. Why? They may make you tired, even in that short period of time.

Paraffin Wax Treatments

Paraffin wax treatments, using melted wax, is a good way to apply heat to the hands. (Make sure you initially use these treatments under the supervision of your doctor or physical therapist.) Usually, the painful area is dipped in melted wax from 10 to 12 times. This forms a very thin, glove-like layer that covers the area, coats it, and keeps it warm for a fairly long period of time. Once the wax is in place, the joint must remain still or else the wax will crack. After anywhere from 15 to 45 minutes, the wax is peeled off. Because of the close adhesion of the wax to the body, it's a good idea *not* to use paraffin treatments on body parts that contain open wounds. It's also important to be very careful while heating the wax, to avoid fire hazards.

Heating Pads

Electric heating pads can be helpful but should not be used for long periods of time. They should be placed on *top* of the painful area. It's not a good idea to lay on a heating pad or sleep with one on. Heating pads are usually safest at low settings.

An electric blanket may also be helpful. Not only does it provide warmth which can be soothing to your joints, but it also means that you'll require fewer blankets in cold weather. So what, you say? Well, if you need fewer blankets, you won't have to bear the weight of a large number of blankets on your already weakened joints! Get it? (CAUTION: Electrical appliances should always be used with discretion.)

Heat Lamps

Heat lamps (diathermy) can be useful for small parts of the body. Infrared bulbs are the best bulbs to use, not ultraviolet bulbs like those found in sunlamps. You want to help your pain, not tan your skin!

Cold

Although there are many benefits to using heat treatments, some people and situations respond better to cold treatment. Cold treatments, also known as cryotherapy, can help painful, inflamed joints due to RA. How? Cold has a numbing effect on nerve endings in the affected areas. It also decreases the activity of the body cells. Furthermore, cold slows the flow of blood. This can be helpful not only in preventing bleeding, but in reducing inflammation.

One common method of cold treatment involves soaking a cloth or towel in ice water, wringing it out and applying it to the painful area. As with hot compresses, it's a good idea to protect yourself, and to prolong the effectiveness of the treatment by using plastic sheets or dry towels. Another type of cold compress can be made by wrapping a towel around a plastic bag that has been filled with ice cubes.

Some people don't like cold treatments, saying they're only good for polar bears. Others, however, may find that greater pain relief can be obtained by using cold rather than heat treatments.

Contrast Baths

Contrast baths may be helpful in relieving pain and swelling for some individuals. You're contrasting hot and cold water treatments. The most common procedure used for contrast baths is to soak the extremities alternately for three minutes in hot water (approximately 110° F) and one minute in cold water (approximately 65° F).

HYDROTHERAPY

Hydrotherapy, or water baths, may be a very helpful way to get your joints more mobile, as well as promoting relaxation, improving deep breathing, increasing circulation, reducing extremity swelling, and improving coordination. Hydrotherapy can also be helpful as a heat technique.

But hydrotherapy can cause fatigue, so it should not be done for a long period of time. And there should be somebody there with you, if possible.

Pool Exercise Programs

Pool exercise programs, also called ''aquatics'' by the Arthritis Foundation, can be very beneficial for your RA. (They can also be helpful if you don't have the disease!) You can exercise many parts of your body in the water. Exercising in pools is safe and much less strenuous than the same exercise outside of the water. It can also be enjoyable! You're more likely to build up the strength of your muscles and range of motion in your joints when you're in the water. It's possible to do much more in water than out of the water. Movements are easier in the water because weight is relieved by its buoyancy. This makes it easier to move joints which are weakened and painful. The warmth tends to reduce the pain and spasms of muscles.

You may find that you feel better about yourself because you're able to move more normally in the water. As a result, you can do more exercise for a longer period of time.

There are many centers that have specific aquatics exercise programs for individuals with arthritis. Check with your local chapter of the Arthritis Foundation for further details.

ALLEVIATING THE PAIN PSYCHOLOGICALLY

Is pain purely physiological? Rarely. It's usually a combination of physiological and psychological factors. What does this mean? Although your joints may be hurting, it's your *mind* that determines just how much they hurt.

Angela was moving exceptionally slowly, primarily because she had a lot of joint pain in her knees. The pain overwhelmed her every time she tried to move faster. Even when she was doing something she enjoyed, her movements were restricted. Suddenly, she heard her 6-year-old son cry out for help. Without thinking about her joint pain, she went flying across the room to help him. This couldn't be purely physiological pain! Yes, Angela was in pain, but her mind had probably magnified it. When she realized that her son was in trouble, her pain temporarily took on secondary importance.

What does all this mean? If medication or other medical intervention doesn't help alleviate your pain, you can still relieve some (if not all) of it by working on your mind's awareness of it. Read on to find out how you can do this.

Relaxation Techniques

Relaxation can be helpful in controlling pain. Relaxation is the opposite of tension, which can actually increase your pain. Relaxation is also helpful in loosening the muscles which may contribute to your pain. There are a number of different types of relaxation procedures including meditation, autogenic training, hypnosis, and deep breathing procedures.

Let's discuss other psychological techniques to help control pain, such as imagery, biofeedback, and changing your way of thinking.

Imagery

There is a relationship between your mind and the way you feel physically. Much research has proven this. Scientists have also found that bodily functions, previously thought to be totally beyond conscious control (autonomic is the scientific term), can be modified using psychological techniques! One such technique is imagery, or the process of conjuring up pictures or scenes in your mind. In practice, imagery has been beneficial in helping to deal with a host of physiological and psychological problems, including headaches, hypertension, depression, and pain. In many cases, imagery procedures have worked well in combination with prescribed medication for treating illness.

Here's how imagery works. Sit in a comfortable chair or in bed and get into a relaxed position. Lights should be dimmed, and outside sounds or noises minimized, with no interruptions. Breathe smoothly and rhythmically, allowing your body to release tension and relax. Then imagine a scene of your own choosing, trying to make the image as vivid and real as possible. This scene can be used therapeutically to help you feel better.

Anita was suffering from a sharp pain in her knees. She was instructed to relax and then develop an image of what this joint pain looked like. She imagined it as a very sharp knife jabbed into her knees. Others may feel like their knees are being hit by a hammer or have dozens of pins stuck into them. Whatever imagery you develop, it should be as vivid and detailed as possible. Anita was then instructed to reverse what was happening in the image: she imagined the knife slowly being removed from the knees, and a soothing cream being applied. Finally, the knife was completely out. She was then able to relax and her discomfort was eliminated.

There are other images you could use to reduce joint pain. For example, you could imagine oil or a soothing lotion being gently massaged on the affected area, or taking a warm bath. These images can be used anywhere. (Have you ever taken a bath on a bus?!) With regular use, they can help you feel better. Imagery is really only restricted by your creativity. A good book on the subject is *In The Mind's Eye* by Arnold Lazarus. See if your public library or local bookstore has it.

Imagery is a key component in hypnosis. Hypnosis can be helpful in RA since it is also quite effective in the area of pain control.

Biofeedback

Biofeedback combines the procedures of relaxation and imagery with the use of measuring instruments—usually electronic ones. These machines let you know what's going on physiologically (giving you *feedback*) in your body (*bio*). The devices, which are connected to different parts of your body, provide moment-by-moment information about any changes that are taking place.

Biofeedback can help you learn to control certain automatic body functions by obtaining feedback from certain measurement techniques. You can learn how to voluntarily control internal functions of your body which you may have previously thought were involuntary or uncontrollable. Blood flow or activities of the brain are among your body's automatic functions.

One of the main advantages of biofeedback is that there are usually signals which you can hear or see. Electrodes are either taped to your skin or attached in some other way. They pick up responses which are transmitted to the biofeedback unit as electrical impulses. These impulses are then translated into sounds or lights that you can observe. In this way, you may receive continuous information about body functions such as blood pressure, heart rate, muscle tension, or skin temperature. Using this information, you can develop different types of imagery so that you can learn how to control your internal responses.

Gayle was experiencing a lot of joint pain in her shoulder, so her physician suggested she try biofeedback. A machine measuring muscle tension was attached to her shoulder (in much the same way that electrodes from an EKG machine are connected. There is *no* pain, and you won't get jolted!). As she attempted to relax, the machine gave her instant feedback as to whether she was really relaxing, and to what degree. As she became aware of her lowering tension, she learned what mental images were helping her to relax. She could then continue using these images on her own, without the machine, to help her relax and control some of the pain.

What kinds of biofeedback equipment may be used? Most frequently, machines can be used to measure skin temperature, pulse, blood pressure, the electrical activity resulting from muscular tension, or electrical activity coming from the brain.

There are some people who wonder whether or not biofeedback does anything other than help you to relax your muscles. Further research is still necessary.

Not much specific research has been done with biofeedback in arthritis. However, research has indicated that biofeedback can be helpful in relaxation training, controlling pain, warming hands, and re-educating muscles. This may be helpful for individuals with RA.

Coping Psychologically

There are other factors that can contribute to the intensity (even the very existence) of your pain, including your emotional state, the attention you pay to it, and the way the rest of your body feels. Obviously, as you pinpoint which of these factors does play a role, you can begin improving the way you cope with pain.

Where do you start? You'll want to do everything you can to decrease fear, stress, tension, and other negative emotional factors. All of these may make you more aware of your painful physical state. Anything you can do to relieve anxiety and tension (including psychotherapy, if necessary) should help you to cope better with any pain.

How do you reduce the amount of attention focused on your pain? Of course, the more time you have to think about it, the worse it will seem. So try to divert your attention. Develop other interests that require concentration. You can always come up with thoughts or activities that will distract you from painful thoughts. One very helpful "activity" might be to get involved with a support group for people living with pain. One such organization is the National Chronic Pain Outreach. They have many chapters throughout the country, and more are always forming. It can be great to know that you're not alone in trying to cope with pain. Who knows? You may even get some great ideas that will help to reduce the pain you have to live with!

AN UNAGONIZING CONCLUSION

If you ever do have any pain, whether from RA, your treatment, or from something else, don't throw in the heating pad! Realize that the pain need not last forever. A lot can be done, both medically and psychologically, to help deal with it.

20

Exercise
(And Rest)

Two of the most important components of any treatment program for RA are rest and exercise. The proper proportion will be determined by your physician specifically for you, since no two people have the same needs.

Let's discuss these two important factors in more detail.

REST

Rest is an important component of treatment for RA. It is necessary to give your joints a chance to "recharge their batteries." It also helps you to maintain an alert, active state.

Because you have RA, regularly-scheduled rest periods may help to keep you as strong as possible for the remainder of your day. However, if you feel very tired too often, this may be your body's way of telling you that you need additional rest periods. So pay attention!

Rest is important. But too much rest can be as dangerous as too little rest. Although inflammation may decrease during rest, rest also allows muscles to become weaker and joints to get stiffer. If you rest too much, your tendons will become weaker and your bones may get even softer. You may feel even more tired. The more rest you get, the more you want, and this creates a vicious cycle.

Rest is vital in learning to live with RA, but it must be properly prescribed. There are differing opinions regarding how long your rest periods should be. Some people feel you should schedule several 5- to 15-minute rest periods per day. Others feel you should schedule two 30- to 60-minute rest periods each day. There are plenty of other opinions, as well. Your physician will help you to determine which rest periods are most appropriate for you. How? By taking into consideration the severity of your disease, your lifestyle, and other aspects of day-to-day living.

If your RA is in a flare, you may need more bed rest (and less exercise) to give your body extra healing time. Hopefully, this additional rest will reduce your pain and inflammation.

EXERCISE

Regular exercise is a very important component of your treatment for RA. Why? The goals of exercise are to build and maintain muscle tone, support and stabilize your joints, reduce fatigue, and maintain or increase mobility. It can also help to prevent some of the deformities that occasionally occur in RA, as well as to improve any joint deformities which may have already occurred. Don't you wish it did all this instantly?

You should try to participate in activities that emphasize good muscle tone, rather than build muscle strength. For example, walking or swimming are better exercises than weight lifting! It's also a good idea to have a regular exercise program, rather than exercising whenever "the spirit moves you!"

Exercise builds strong bones. How? When you exercise, your body absorbs more calcium. This calcium finds its way to your bones, causing them to become thicker and sturdier. Muscles also grow stronger and become better toned as a result of exercise. This helps to stabilize and strengthen your joints. Exercise strengthens tendons and ligaments, also important for joint stability. All these body parts become weaker when they're not used often enough.

Bones do not have their own blood supply. But oxygen and nourishment get to the bone as a result of fluid being squeezed into the joint space. How to squeeze? You got it—exercise! The motion of exercise is a very important factor in determining the health of your cartilage.

Exercise is also essential to keeping your body trim. You'll want to keep your muscles firm, firm, firm—which is better than flab, flab, flab! Exercise can also help your body systems to work efficiently.

But remember the need for a proper balance between rest and exercise. Too much exercise may increase the pain and inflammation in your joints, doing more harm than good. This proper balance can best be determined by your physician or other health professionals. However, only by trial-and-error can you really determine whether you are exercising or resting in the proper amounts.

Is Exercise Good Only For Your Body?

Exercise is as important for psychological well-being as it is for your body. Exercise gives you the feeling of being able to do something. It can build up your self-confidence. Have you lost some good feelings about yourself due to your medical condition and the way it has changed your body image? Exercise can help. It will restore some confidence to your body. Seeing improvement in your performance as a result of exercise can also build up your self-esteem. Exercise clears your mind, keeps you alert, and helps to control some of the unpleasant emotional reactions that may occur from time to time. Exercise can help to control stress, as well as emotions such as depression, anger, fear, and frustration.

Exercise can help you to enjoy deep sleep, so you'll feel better the next day. And unless you exercise alone, you'll enjoy some healthy social interactions—always good for the mind (as well as the body)!

Exercise for Children

Exercise is a very important part of JRA treatment to keep joints mobile and prevent disabilities or deformity. It's important for the child, parents, and physician to work together in order to determine the amount of activity that's appropriate.

Exercise can be helpful either in a planned exercise regimen or in simple play activities. Although it may be necessary for children to get up a little earlier in the morning, exercise can help them to loosen up before school.

The child with JRA may even need to walk around in the classroom from time to time in order to avoid joint stiffness. This may have to be explained to the teacher and other children in the class.

Muscle tone and mobility in children with JRA can be helped with exercise programs and physical therapy.

Getting Started

Your exercise program will be designed especially for you! (Aren't you lucky?) It will be prepared by your physician, physical therapist, occupational therapist, or any combination of these professionals. The specifics of your exercise program will depend upon the severity of your RA, the severity of your pain and inflammation, your overall physical condition, and the joints affected.

If your medical condition has kept you from being active, be prepared for something frustrating. When you first begin to exercise again, *wow,* will you be out of shape! That's not a put-down. Your muscles will need time to regain their strength. So any kind of exercise should be implemented gradually. The longer it's been since you've done any exercising, the slower your return should be. To benefit most from an exercise program, you must do it regularly.

Exercising Caution

Make sure you have your doctor's approval before proceeding. Then start building up your exercise ability gradually. Don't exceed the moderation that's required.

You'll want to learn the difference between muscle soreness (which is a normal response to exercise) and increased joint pain (which may mean that either you're overdoing it, or you're participating in an exercise that's a no-no).

Be careful with your exercise. If you exercise an inflamed joint, the inflammation may temporarily worsen. Therefore, although exercise doesn't necessarily have to stop if your joints are inflamed, it should either focus on joints which aren't affected, or very carefully (and minimally) on joints that are.

It's probably not a good idea to participate in high-tension exercises, such as weight lifting or ball squeezing. Nor should you become involved in "jerky" sports such as tennis, bowling, or golf. Not only do these require strength that you may not have, but they may put too much immediate pressure on joints that you don't want to stress. Another example is bicycling. If RA is causing your knees to become sore or swollen, it makes sense not to bicycle, since it can be very stressful on your knees.

Categories of Exercise

What are you trying to accomplish through exercise? That usually determines how to categorize it. In other words, exercise can be divided into range of motion, stretching, muscle strengthening, and endurance (or functional) exercises.

Range of Motion

A joint's normal movements (in different directions) fall into the category "range of motion." RA may sometimes reduce the range of motion possible in a particular joint. So exercise attempts to stop that reduction. Just as importantly, it tries to gradually increase the range of motion that is possible.

Range of motion exercises stretch joints in various directions by manipulating the muscles attached to them. Range of motion exercises that are involved in RA may be very helpful in preventing loss of motion, restoring lost movement, and reducing stiffness. Range of motion exercises help you to maintain normal movement in your joints. Finally, range of motion exercises try to prevent any deformity in the joints.

Strengthening Exercises

Some exercises are important because they build up strength in the muscles or other tissues that support the joints and keep them stable. These exercises also help maintain the strength that you already have.

There are two types of strengthening (or muscle-tightening) exercises which may be helpful to you. Isometric exercises are strengthening exercises which do not involve any movement within the joints. You strongly tighten the muscle but do not move the joint. As a result, strength can be improved without further stressing the joints. Resistive exercises actively move the joint against a resistance, such as a weight, or against other objects. Because there is less chance of stressing an already-fragile joint, isometric exercises are usually considered safer than resistive exercises.

Positioning or Stretching Exercises

Positioning exercises can be very important, especially in RA. Hips, knees, hands, and shoulders are particularly vulnerable to stiffness and deformity in RA. By stretching your body into certain positions, you may be able to help yourself avoid some of these deformities. Examples of positioning exercises include reaching a high spot on the door, or stretching out on your bed.

Stretching exercises are done to relieve any stiffness or tightness in the muscles or tendons surrounding a joint. If pain immobilizes a joint, the muscles controlling that joint are not doing anything. This disuse will adversely affect the muscle, causing such problems as spasms, cramps, or decreased flexibility. Stretching exercises can help that problem.

Endurance Exercises

Endurance exercises are also referred to as aerobic exercises. These are less beneficial for specific joints but more helpful for overall fitness. They are usually a good complement to range of motion and strengthening exercises. Examples of exercises for endurance are walking, swimming, and bicycling. Endurance exercises build up heart and lung strength. They can also reduce chronic fatigue and improve overall physical fitness.

Active vs. Passive Exercises

Another way of categorizing exercise is as either active or passive. If you're moving your body without anybody else helping you, you're doing active exercises. If you're moving it and someone is helping you, these are active assistive exercises. If you "relax" while a physical therapist, family member, or friend moves your joints (for example, if you're in a severe flare), then you're doing passive exercises.

Guidelines for Exercise Benefits

To be sure you derive the best benefits from an exercise program, there are certain guidelines you should follow:

• Don't feel that you have to wait until you feel better before starting your exercise program. Starting sooner may even help you to feel better more quickly. But get professional advice and supervision.

• Develop your ability to tolerate exercises slowly. Because one goal of exercise programs is to improve the functioning of your joints and muscles, keep trying to increase the amount of exercise you do, but do this gradually. Too rapid an increase, or too intense an exercise program, may only increase the pain that you're experiencing. It may also damage the very joint that you want to protect and improve.

• If you experience a lot of pain or inflammation in your joints, exercise must be done with much more caution. Isometric exercises may be helpful. Very gentle range of motion exercises may also be suggested.

• Anticipate minor discomfort from exercising. Remember, you're moving joints that may not want to be moved! Bending a joint and stretching the surrounding muscles, tendons, and ligaments may cause some pain. It's actually a good idea to push a joint a little beyond the level at which pain first occurs. This helps to increase joint mobility and prevents contractures! Applying heat before exercising may help to relax tense muscles, reducing pain. But if you experience too much discomfort or pain, or if it lasts for a long time, cut back. It may indicate that you're overdoing!

•Aim to do as much exercise as possible on your own, even though you may initially need help in doing your exercises—either from a family member or a physical therapist.

•Don't compare your exercise program to somebody else's. You wouldn't compare your doses or types of medication to somebody else's, would you? (Or should you?)

21

Surgery

Not too many people cherish the thought of "going under the knife." Even so, surgery is considered to be one of the more recent and successful methods of treatment for RA, and can certainly affect your lifestyle.

When can surgery be helpful? If other approaches (such as medication, rest, physical therapy, and other preventive measures) fail to alleviate pain or reduce disability or deformity, then surgery may be considered as an alternative procedure. However, most arthritis experts recommend trying all other modalities first before considering surgery. If RA is severe enough, causing irreparable damage to the joints or other tissues surrounding the joints, surgery may be necessary. It can be a very effective way to return to a more satisfactory, active life.

The most likely result of surgery is relief from pain. In addition, it can restore comfort and mobility to joints affected by RA. It can also be useful in correcting serious deformities.

Surgery is usually an elective procedure. Although you may feel you need it because of pain or disability, it's usually not something that is done on an emergency basis.

WHY SURGERY?

If joint cartilage is worn away as a result of RA, the joints may become painful, stiff, or weak and unstable. If this damage becomes severe, excruciating pain, loss of function, and deformity may result. If RA damages a tendon, the joint may be much less functional—if not totally immobilized.

Weight-bearing joints may be affected to the point where you have great difficulty walking. If your disease seriously affects your upper extremities, you may find that you're barely able to perform even the simplest activities of daily living.

WHO CAN BENEFIT?

Surgical procedures can currently be used on individuals of virtually any age, although surgery is usually less desirable for younger individuals. Surgery is usually not a treatment of choice in JRA unless the condition has severely restricted mobility. Surgery is rarely considered early in JRA development.

WHY NOT SURGERY?

If surgery can do so much good, why isn't it appropriate for everyone? Unfortunately, RA surgery is not a cure! It may help the symptoms, but it won't eliminate the condition. However, even though surgery can't cure the illness, at least it can significantly relieve many of the problems that come with it. Surgery may be less effective in RA than in other types of arthritis (like osteoarthritis, for example. Osteoarthritis usually affects only one or a few joints, whereas RA usually attacks several. It would become more difficult to start replacing several affected joints.)

Surgery can be painful and expensive, and it can require a long recovery period. It also keeps you away from certain activities that you may normally enjoy. You may argue, though, that your condition before surgery prevented you from doing these things, anyway. Another problem with surgery is that it's not always successful, although the success rates have been increasing dramatically. If you have a heart condition or lung disease (or other problems exist), surgery may be contraindicated, since it may pose a higher risk for you even if the outcome is positive.

TYPES OF SURGERY

In determining what type of surgery is done, the orthopedic surgeon must consider several factors, including your condition, the joints affected, the degree to which your joints have been affected, and your age and lifestyle.

Arthroplasty

An increasingly common surgical procedure for rheumatoid arthritis is arthroplasty. This refers to any surgical procedure which restructures a joint.

There are two types of arthroplasty. In one, parts of a damaged joint surface are removed. A surgical reformation, or shaping, of the joint can help to rebuild damaged joints. In this procedure, the ends of the bone where cartilage has worn away are resurfaced or relined. This eliminates the problem of bone or ligament damage due to cartilage erosion. Arthroplasty may actually create a false joint, where only some of the bone in the joint may be removed or the bones may be realigned.

There's a problem with this, however. Although a partial restoration may restore some function, pain is still possible. The joint may still prove to be unstable if it's a weight-bearing joint. The trend today seems to be away from these partial resolutions to the problem and towards total joint replacement.

The second type of arthroplasty is joint replacement. In joint replacement surgery the old joint is removed and replaced by an artificial one (a prosthesis), usually constructed of plastic and metal. This is probably the most dramatic and exciting surgical procedure for RA.

Total joint replacement for the hip and knees are the most frequent (and successful) arthroplasty operations. Shoulder replacement is becoming more successful, as is knuckle replacement. Research continues on surgery for replacement of the wrist, ankle, and elbow.

Joint replacement surgery usually isn't done with children until the child has stopped growing. As a result, it usually isn't considered until the child is 16 or older. A lot of preparation is necessary for this surgery from a psychological point of view. Why? Because the life of the artificial replacement is such that additional surgery may be necessary in the future.

Let's Get Hip

The hip joint is the largest joint in the body. It's also one of the most important weight-bearing joints. A problem in this joint can certainly affect you. The hip joint can become rigid and unusable. The pain may make any kind of movement almost impossible.

Several thousand total hip replacements are done each year. It has gotten to the point where hip replacements are considered almost routine surgery—successful more than 95% of the time.

Synovectomy

Another surgical procedure for RA is the synovectomy. The joint is opened, and part or all of the diseased synovial membrane is removed. Why? Because the inflammation in the synovial membrane causes it to thicken and spread out. Then, release of enzymes damages the nearby cartilage, bone, and tendons. Usually, a synovectomy is done in cases where joint inflammation is severe and irreversible. It's also important that the joint be fairly easily within reach, such as in the fingers or knees.

There's a problem, though. Frequently, even after the synovial membrane has been removed, it grows back. When that happens, any pain or swelling that occurred before may return.

A synovectomy isn't performed as frequently on children as it used to be. The more commonly-used procedure in children is called a capsulotomy. If a child with JRA suffers muscle contractures, the capsulotomy may be considered. This is also called a soft tissue release. It may help to improve the positioning of a joint that has been deformed by chronic contractures. This procedure involves cutting the tissues that cause the contracture, allowing the joint to return to a more normal position.

Arthrodesis

Another procedure used is called arthrodesis, or surgical fusion. Two bones may be fused together to stabilize or strengthen a weak joint. Although the bones in this joint will no longer be able to move (because the fusion freezes them rigidly in place), at least the joint will be able to support weight more easily and without pain.

Surgical fusion may be used, for example, at the joint at the base of your thumb. This can help to restore at least some degree of mobility to your hand—mobility which may have been lost due to pain and restrictions.

Arthrodesis may also be done on your spine. If inflammation from RA causes your vertebrae to become wobbly and unstable, this may threaten your spinal cord, which could seriously damage (or even paralyze) your body.

Arthrodesis is now used more commonly on the wrist, the fingers, the ankle, the toes, and top vertebrae in the neck. For other joints, joint replacement may be more desirable.

Osteotomy

The osteotomy is a procedure which attempts to correct a deformity in a joint. One of the two bones in the joint is cut and reset in a better alignment. Why is this done? If the cartilage on one bone is worn away more than the other, the result is a bad bone alignment in the joint. After the osteotomy, the bones will be in a better position.

Resection

A resection is another surgical procedure where part of a bone, or all of it, is removed. This is usually done in situations where the removal of the bone or joint will not significantly affect mobility. Resection procedures are often done with the metatarsal joint in the feet when it's too painful or difficult to walk. Resection of the end of the ulna bone in the wrist can help reduce pain and deformity of that joint.

Arthroscopy

Arthroscopy is a relatively new surgical procedure. It makes use of a small periscope-type instrument (the arthroscope) to look into the joint. The arthroscope, which is a little bit wider than a drinking straw, enables the surgeon to see practically everything that's inside the joint. The arthroscope can be useful in diagnosing problems within a joint.

Bits of torn bone or cartilage can be shaved or removed during this procedure. Joints may be cleaned out. A partial synovectomy can be done through the arthroscope, too. Little pieces of bone or cartilage which may be floating freely in the joint fluid can be removed during surgery. Arthroscopy is most commonly used on the knee, but can also be used on the hip and shoulder.

An older procedure in which the joint is exposed to allow diagnosis or repair is called arthrotomy. This procedure isn't done as often since the advent of arthroscopy.

Tendon Repair

Surgical procedures to repair tendons may also be done if RA has affected the fingers or hand. In these cases, the disease may cause the outer surface of the bone to fray. The tendon sheath may tear. In tendon repair procedures, the damaged bone surface may be removed. Damaged tissue is repaired, and weakened tissue is tightened up and attached to healthy tissue nearby.

WHAT HAPPENS AFTER SURGERY?

After surgery, it's time for rehabilitation. Your program will include rest, physical therapy, and gradually-increasing amounts of activity. You'll need plenty of rest. You'll also need time to get used to assistive devices such as crutches, canes, or splints, to support the surgically-repaired or replaced joints during this phase. You'll probably learn special exercises so you can regain strength and mobility in whatever joint was involved in surgery. (By the way, exercise rehabilitation is good before surgery, too, to make the after-surgery rehabilitation a bit easier.)

Be careful. You don't want to take a chance of damaging the joint that has just been repaired! In all probability, it will take at least a few weeks before you can resume your usual routine. You may want to make arrangements to have somebody help out at home for a while following surgery.

THINGS TO THINK ABOUT

Surgery can result in an abrupt change in your condition. It may be permanent or temporary. But there are certainly some important things for you to think about.

• Ask yourself a very simple question: "Will the surgery make a big difference in the quality of my lifestyle?" If so, fine. Continue to consider it. But if not, why consider it at all?

• Here's something else to be aware of. Although pain can be relieved and a good degree of mobility may be restored, it doesn't mean that you'll be able to get involved in professional football or other strenuous physical activities! Yes, you'll be able to do more, but there'll be differences between what you can do with artificial joints and what you were able to do with the healthy joints you had before developing RA.

• Get a second opinion. This is always important before deciding whether or not surgery is the treatment for you.

• Ask your primary physician for recommendations regarding who should perform the surgery. You'll probably want an orthopedic surgeon for joint replacement surgery. If surgery is being done on your hand, for example, you'll probably want a specialist in hand surgery. Your surgeon should be someone you feel comfortable with and who also has extensive experience in exactly the type of surgery you need.

- •Discuss what's involved in the operation, and what kind of rehabilitation will follow. What will you need to know before, during, and after the procedure? Feel free to ask questions. Remember: Preparation for surgery makes the outcome easier to handle!

- •Prepare yourself for extensive rehabilitation after surgery. In almost all cases, successful surgery depends not only on the surgery itself, but on the diligence with which you participate in rehabilitation *following* the surgery.

22

Quackery

Elaine was frustrated. She had been taking medication for months to relieve her RA pain. Although her pain was somewhat diminished, she still wasn't able to do what she wanted to do. Doctors consistently told her there was nothing else that could be done for her at this point. Therefore, her eyes lit up when she read an advertisement for a "cure" for RA. Without thinking twice, she wrote out a check for $39.95 and mailed it to the "pharmaceutical" company that described a particular nutritional supplement which was guaranteed "to relieve your arthritis symptoms in less than 30 days, or your money back."

Three weeks later she received the small vial of bitter-tasting pills. When she had finished all the pills after 30 days, she realized that not only had her physical pain remained the same (fortunately, she had continued to follow her physician-prescribed treatment program), but she also had the added mental anguish of knowing that she had been duped!

When you're dealing with something as long-lasting and uncomfortable as RA, it's important that your illness be treated properly. But what if you become impatient with your treatment? What if it doesn't seem to bring about results as quickly as you'd like? You may become tempted if somebody suggests a particular technique or item that is the "latest miracle cure!" This is known as the lure of "quackery."

WHAT IS QUACKERY?

Quack remedies are treatments which are fraudulent because they do not have a scientific basis. They do not have a sufficient amount of scientific evidence to prove their effectiveness. In other words, there is no reason to believe that they will work and, in all probability, no real evidence that they do! These quack techniques are usually promoted to the public in an extravagant way. Your vulnerability is what's at stake, and whoever is hawking the technique is taking advantage of that.

Where did the term "quack" come from? In the 17th century, the term "quacksalver" was used to describe a charlatan who bragged that certain products had magic curative powers. These phonies didn't know anything about medicine or about their patients. The term "quack" is an abbreviation for quacksalver.

Not all quacks are blatantly cruel people. Some people really and truly believe that their techniques work and are really trying to help people. In some cases, remedies may even be advocated by doctors and it may be hard to differentiate or distinguish these from legitimate treatments. However, you still want to be wary. You don't want to be the unsuccessful guinea pig who eventually learns that such techniques are not valid!

HOW MUCH DOES QUACKERY COST?

Unfortunately, billions of dollars are spent each year on quack remedies and devices. This has become a very serious problem (except for the quack!). And here's another mind-boggler: For every $1 that is spent on legitimate and appropriate scientific treatment for RA, more than $25 is spent on quack remedies, phony pain relievers, and inappropriate cures!

WHO'S SUSCEPTIBLE TO QUACKERY?

If you've been experiencing never-ending pain, increasing disability, and problems with (or deformity of) your joints, you may be vulnerable. If you feel that your physician is less able to do the most desirable job, you might find yourself susceptible to the promises of a quack.

Don't be ashamed to admit that you've been approached by, or even considered buying from, a quack. Virtually anybody who has been affected by RA has been taken in at least once. (I won't ask if you're one of them—those sheepish grins give me the answer!) Consider yourself lucky, however, if you recognized your mistake early enough and were able to avoid being taken for a ride.

So why do so many people fall victims to quackery? The quack promises a quick, easy cure for a long-term problem. You already know that traditional treatment programs for RA do not work overnight and that you have to adhere strictly to them in order for them to work. In some cases, especially when you're most vulnerable, it's simply too hard to pass up! You may figure, "What do I have to lose?" (A lot!)

HOW CAN QUACKERY HURT YOU?

What will you lose if you try a quack remedy? Besides money, there are a number of things that you may lose. You may also lose patience, confidence, dignity, courage and, in certain extreme cases, life!

Money can be a problem. Although it may only cost you a few dollars for a book or copper bracelet, it can get more expensive when fraudulent programs of injections or spa treatments are involved. These may cost up to thousands of dollars. Remember, a quack isn't in the business for ego-building or gratification, A quack does it for the money!

Quackery may convince you to forego standard medical treatment. If this happens, you won't derive appropriate benefits from whatever medical treatment can be helpful to you. There is also the danger that the quack approach may cause additional damage. This may occur if the quack treatment actually covers up further deterioration of your joints.

Trying a quack approach is not only financially draining, it's also psychologically draining. You build up your hopes that something is going to work, and when it doesn't, you feel even worse than you did before. This disillusionment can certainly undermine your courage and determination to live with your condition. Your patience may be sorely tested. You may find it even more difficult to participate in an appropriate treatment program.

It can be terrible to lose your dignity. You may feel ripped off, or that somebody took advantage of you. Your integrity and pride have been damaged. Don't continue to feel this way. Write off what you've done. Accept the fact that you were zonked and move on to more appropriate treatment.

EXAMPLES OF QUACKERY

The different types of quack techniques may be divided into three categories: drugs, diets, and devices. What are some examples of miracle cures with little validity? Consider some of the following:

Drugs: Indian medicines, vitamin injections, iodine

Diets: Immunized "milk," alfalfa seeds, crow's meat, gelatin, seaweed, worms, yogurt, fish oils, mineral waters, fasting, eating only uncooked foods, eating only cooked foods

Devices: Copper bracelets, electric belts, magic horse collars, magnetic devices, zinc disks, teeth extractions, mistletoe, polyvinyl clothing, special underwear, sulfur baths, applications of a hot poker, electric shocks, sitting for prolonged periods in abandoned uranium mines

A Little More Detail, Please

Many of the quack remedies are based on changes in diet. Keep in mind that extensive research has indicated that, other than eating to keep healthy, no major diet problems have either prevented or exacerbated arthritic problems.

Whenever you read of a "diet to cure arthritis," you should be a little skeptical. Why? The key word is "cure." At the present time, RA cannot be cured. In some cases, these diets may be more damaging because they may not provide you with the nutrients or fluids you need for a balanced, healthy diet. Research hasn't shown any indication that a specialized diet can play a role in helping RA. Therefore, when an individual says that a particular ingredient will make your RA go away, it's something to beware of.

Venoms are often advocated as ways to cure arthritis. Venoms coming from animals or insects such as snakes, ants, or bees have been touted as being the miracle cure for RA. What's the bite? What if you're allergic to these venoms? You might experience reactions that are even more serious than RA itself!

Some people believe that wearing copper bracelets can be helpful because the chemical nature of the copper can alleviate a deficiency within the body. The answer to this is simple: If you enjoy wearing a copper bracelet, and you feel it's attractive and adds to your looks, fine. But don't expect it to result in significant changes in your RA.

Certain clinics may also fall under the quack category if they promise miraculous cures costing a mere several thousand dollars. It is true that in these days you get what you pay for. This may cause the unwary individual to believe that paying a lot of money increases the likelihood of success. Promoters are aware of this, and will milk you as much as they can.

PROTECT YOURSELF!

With all of the unproven methods and quack remedies promoted in magazines, books, or through different individuals, how do you know which are real and which aren't? It's hard to decide if a remedy is really quackery—especially if, while using a quack remedy, you go into remission! But was it the quack remedy that was responsible for the remission? Or could it be the "placebo effect," in which your strong belief in what you were taking or doing helped produce the desired effect? Or might this have happened anyway due to your regular treatment program, or a spontaneous remission? What if the disease returns later in full force? If you're convinced that the quack treatment did cause the remission, dependence on it may prove extremely dangerous.

How can you protect yourself from quacks or their remedies? Before trying anything, investigate it carefully. Be suspicious. Be cautious. Speak to your own physician. You should even be aware of other individuals who may claim to be physicians to try to convince you that they have a cure for RA. Check with The Arthritis Foundation, the Food and Drug Administration, or even with The National Institute of Health.

There is a problem with checking with your physician. In many cases, physicians are so busy that they may not be aware of, or understand, the technique that the quack is trying to push. This may confirm, in your mind, what the quack has been saying all along: that the medical profession disregards the needs of the person with arthritis and doesn't have time to investigate all the possibilities. This may bother you, and may make you more vulnerable to what the quack is saying. The quacks know this. That's why they're using this argument in the first place! Don't let that cause you to doubt your physician. There may still be good reasons to reject the idea that the quack is trying to sell you on.

Although some quack remedies may seem harmless, they can still hurt you if they keep you from following an appropriate treatment program for rheumatoid arthritis. Keep that in mind. Try not to let anyone convince you that you should no longer follow an appropriate treatment. If you have questions about whether your doctor is prescribing the treatment that's best for you, it's better to get a second opinion from another physician than from a quack!

BEWARE OF THE "RED FLAGS!"

What should you beware of? Any of the following could be a give-away that the remedy is quackery:

- Beware of any procedure which promises quick, easy relief of pain.

- Beware of any treatment program that advocates a special diet or nutritional approach as the answer to rheumatoid arthritis.

•Beware of any secret formulas, devices, or programs which will "cure" rheumatoid arthritis. At the present time, there is no cure for RA. If any kind of miraculous discovery were made, you would be sure to learn about it in the newspaper, on the evening news, or from some other reputable source.

•Beware of quacks who claim that their cure or remedy is exclusive or secret. You might ask them why, if it does such a good job at helping so many people, an honest person would keep it a secret? Or ask them why you didn't hear about it through a more appropriate channel! Scientists who are legitimately a part of the medical world do not keep such discoveries exclusive or secret.

•Beware of any technique that has no scientific proof of its safety and effectiveness. Keep in mind that the promoter probably hasn't had any kind of clinical trials to test the method.

•Beware of anything that is advocated in a rag magazine or tabloid, through a mail promotion, or by somebody that you meet in a store or at a meeting.

•Beware of any advertisements which offer testimonials or case histories of individuals who are satisfied with a particular program or approach. If somebody indeed finds an answer to helping people with arthritis, it will not be necessary to advertise.

•Beware of anyone who starts off claiming that they know exactly what you're going through, what symptoms you're experiencing, and then explain how they're going to help cleanse your body of any poisons it may contain.

•Beware of anybody who attacks the standard medical treatment of rheumatoid arthritis or who states that appropriate medical procedures (such as drugs or surgery) are unnecessary because they're damaging and dangerous. This may include allegations that medical professionals are deliberately withholding treatment approaches that can be more helpful. Some quacks may accuse the medical profession of trying to interfere with attempts to get their remedy approved. Frequently, these attacks will be launched toward The Arthritis Foundation, The Food and Drug Administration, or even The American Medical Association.

•Beware of the efforts of friends or family to persuade you to try a quack approach. This may be harder to resist than if it were to come from a stranger. Your family and friends really want you to feel better. They don't like to see you suffer and are only too eager to find some kind of solution to your problem. This may make *them* ripe and vulnerable to a quack's suggestions, which they'll then pressure you to try. Now not only will you have to resist the remedy, but you may also have to conquer the guilt that may arise ("Why won't you try this, dear? Don't you want to help yourself?")!

THE FINAL QUACK UP

It's always important to do the best you can to help yourself. You definitely want to feel better, and you want treatment to do the best it can to help you. You don't want to waste time, money, or psychological energy on quack remedies. Always aim to do the best you can to help yourself, but appropriately!

23

Financial Problems

Having RA can be a pain in the pocketbook! Any chronic illness can be expensive, and RA is no exception. The cost of having arthritis ranges up to the billions of dollars in the United States. However, the cost of living with RA that is the most devastating is the human cost: the pain and suffering that must be endured.

Why are the financial costs so high? The cost of treatment and other medical costs, as well as the cost of medication, physical therapy, or other rehabilitative therapies, all add up. Medical costs build as a result of doctor's visits, laboratory tests, physical or occupational therapy, drugs, surgery, support devices, transportation, counseling sessions, and homemakers' services. In addition, money is lost from the number of work days that are missed because of symptoms. And there are other expenses, too. How about the billions of dollars that are spent on quack remedies? The cost (and source) for each person with RA varies considerably. It doesn't take long for financial security to drain into a financial problem.

INSURANCE CAN BE AN ASSURANCE

Fortunately, some people can have some of their costs defrayed by insurance. Insurance coverage is essential. For individuals with RA, certain costs may be reimbursable by third-party payments. Insurance companies do cover a number of medical costs. But what happens if you run out of money or insurance, or if your coverage is not good enough? Because you have a chronic illness, you may have more difficulty getting either life or health insurance. Speak to a reputable insurance agent and find out exactly what you are entitled to. Also speak with a social worker to learn what your community offers in the way of aid.

WORK OR HOME

Financial problems arise from lost earnings or income. You may not be able to work at all, or perhaps you can only hold down a part-time job. Your condition may affect your ability to work. This may cause problems with your job. So it's possible that your "employability" will be reduced because of your RA. Rheumatoid arthritis can also be costly because of changes at home. You may need to have other people help you, or you may need to make renovations in your home. You may need help around the house, such as a babysitter or a cleaning person. All of these things cost money, adding to your financial burden. As your medical costs rise, your budget becomes tighter and tighter. If costs continue to skyrocket, you may feel like you're being strangled!

CAN ANYTHING HELP?

Although RA can be an expensive disease, it need not be alarmingly so—if you're careful. If you take proper care of yourself and begin treatment as early as possible, you can prevent more serious (and expensive) problems from arising.

The use of generic medication can save you money. Generic medication is sold by its chemical name rather than a more common brand name. Ask your physician if it's acceptable to take generic medication. (Remember—not all generics work as well as brand name medication.) You can also save money by refusing to shell out great amounts of money for quack remedies.

If medical costs are overwhelming you, consider attending a clinic. Because clinics usually operate on a sliding-scale fee schedule, you may be able to get quality medical care at a reduced cost. In some cases, you may even see the same physician you'd normally see, since many physicians graciously donate their time to clinics.

If you have questions about financial problems, you may want to check with either The Arthritis Foundation or the Department of Social Services. They may be able to provide you with information and resources and, in some cases, provide emergency assistance. The Arthritis Foundation can tell you which benefits you may be qualified for and how to apply for them.

So before you do anything, talk to people. Find out what others have done. How do you find them? Ask your physician or nurse for suggestions, or contact your local chapter of The Arthritis Foundation for ideas. Speak to others in similar situations to find out how they handle their money problems. Even though you may initially be embarrassed to bring up the subject, the common bond that exists among people with RA tends to smooth this over rather quickly. You'll be glad you brought it up!

UNCLE SAM TO THE RESCUE

Some government insurance programs may be very important sources of financial support. You may be covered (at least to some degree) by Medicare, where eligibility is determined by age, chronic disability, or both; Medicaid, where benefits vary from state to state; or social security disability insurance. Let's discuss these different government programs, what they do, and how you can participate (if you're eligible).

Social Security (Disability)

If you are unable to work because of your RA, you may be eligible for disability benefits. However, you may experience all kinds of legal problems because of the many different definitions of disability.

The Social Security Disability Program is a Federal Government Program. It is administered and run by the Social Security Administration. The money that funds the Social Security Benefit Plan comes from workers and their employers. Because of this, one of the main requirements for receiving benefits is that you must have worked for five out of the ten years prior to your disability. However, if you became disabled before turning 31, the five-year requirement is reduced to one and a half years. In other words, if Ursula Unabletowork, age 28, wanted to receive disability benefits, she would only have to prove that she worked for eighteen months during the previous ten years. However, if Ursula was lying (to herself and the government) about her age and was actually 38, she'd then have to prove five years of work experience in the past ten.

Benefits are available from the Social Security Disability Program to those of you who fit into the following categories:

1. Individuals under the age of 22 who were disabled before that age and are still disabled.
2. Widows who are disabled.
3. Widowers who are disabled and also dependent.

There are also other specific cases that may entitle you to benefits.

There is one very rigid rule that the Social Security Administration enforces in order for benefits to be approved. This guideline is: "The physical or mental impairment must prevent you from doing any substantial, gainful work, and is expected to last (or has lasted) for at least twelve months, or is expected to result in death." In other words, it is expected that your disability prevents you from doing any meaningful work. This must be the case if you are applying for disability benefits.

Once you meet the eligibility requirements for disability benefits, does that mean that cash will start pouring in? Not so fast! There are still other steps that you have to go through. You'll have to provide the names and addresses of people involved in treating you, including physicians, hospitals, or clinics. Medical records must be provided, substantiating the dates and treatments prescribed. This information will be evaluated by a Social Security team (including a physician), and additional tests may be required to support your claim.

Supplemental Security Income (SSI)

Once you apply for Social Security benefits, you also become eligible for Supplemental Security Income. This leads to eligibility for Medicaid. The Supplementary Security Income Program is also run by the Social Security Administration, which operates the Social Security Benefit Program. However, whereas Social Security benefits come from workers and their employers, SSI comes from a general treasury fund.

SSI benefits are available to individuals 65 and over, the blind, and the disabled. The requirements to receive SSI include the same definitions of disability that are used for Social Security benefits.

Medicaid

Medicaid is the more commonly-used term for Medical Assistance. Benefits are provided automatically for anyone who qualifies for Supplemental Security Income. Medicaid will cover virtually any medical-related expense, as long as you go to a professional who is a "participant provider." This provider is then directly reimbursed by the state for the service provided to you.

Medicaid applies if you are 65 or over and are receiving Social Security, or if you are under 65 and have met the Social Security requirements for disability. In addition, Medicaid is provided to families on welfare, and to children under age 21.

Medicare

Medicare is another part of the Social Security Administration. There are two components to the Medicare Program. The medical insurance component helps you to pay for physicians' services and out-patient services, including physical therapy and speech pathology. The hospital insurance component covers in-patient care and nursing care within a facility.

Medicare benefits are limited and rigidly evaluated. They are only applied to charges that are deemed reasonable and necessary in treating your disease. In order to be eligible for Medicare benefits, you must have received disability checks for at least two consecutive years.

HOW ABOUT CHILDREN?

Children affected by JRA may be eligible for financial assistance with medical or educational problems through the Crippled Children's Services, the Developmental Disabilities Act, or under Public Law 94-142.

WHAT SHOULD YOU DO?

To determine whether or not any of these programs are applicable to you, contact your local Social Security office. In addition, consult your physician or your local support groups. These sources should provide you with valuable information that will assist you in determining which programs can help you. But beware. These programs are strict. They are more eager (so it seems) to reject your claim than to accept it. You can appeal if your application is rejected, but this becomes even more aggravating. Want some advice? Talk to people who have been through it. Talk with members of your local support groups. Fight for your rights—and for your dollars.

$UMMING UP

Although RA can be costly, there's still some hope. More and more people are learning about its costly impact. Hopefully, the variety of insurance coverages available to you will increase, more provisions will be made for meeting your expenses, and requirements and application procedures will become more "human."

24

Traveling

Eddie was a 42-year-old car salesman. One reason why he always enjoyed working hard at his job was because it provided him with an income sufficient to take his family on luxurious annual vacations. He and his family would spend many happy weeks in many different parts of the world. However, since he was diagnosed with RA, Eddie had not taken any trips at all. Why? You see, Eddie was afraid that his pain would interfere with his sightseeing plans, so he didn't want to go at all. Need it be this way? Definitely not. Very few restrictions need to be placed on your travel plans. As a matter of fact, you can probably go just about anywhere!

If you think you might like to travel, discuss it with your physician first. Chances are, if you're able to get around your own neighborhood without assistance, you can probably handle traveling with confidence. If you do have difficulty getting around, you'll want to be more selective in where you go. Some people opt to use wheelchairs to protect joints as well as increase the distance they can travel. That might not be a bad idea. But others are afraid of being seen in a wheelchair, or are even more afraid that once they use them, they'll be stuck in them forever. Neither of these fears is valid, but both can interfere with happy travel plans. Work on them.

Do all individuals with RA avoid traveling? No. Some don't travel simply because they feel it's too expensive. This may have nothing to do with RA. But plenty of others do travel, whether their trips are short or long. Some travel simply to prove to themselves that they can. This doesn't mean that there are no fears attached. But they do want to prove to themselves that they can do it, and that traveling, as one of life's pleasures, is possible. As with any other aspect of living with your RA, planning ahead and taking the proper precautions can allow you to travel with a free mind (although not with free airfare!).

What types of planning ahead should you do before a vacation? Let's explore some of them.

When making hotel reservations or other accommodations, make sure that they fit your needs. You'll want to know where you can get proper medical care if necessary. So prepare for this. Write out a list of clinics, hospitals, and physicians in different parts of the world where you may be traveling. In addition, find out if there is a local chapter of the Arthritis Foundation at your destination. This can be very comforting to know.

TAKING MEDICATION AND OTHER SUPPLIES

One of your biggest concerns about traveling may be: What happens if I run out of sufficient medication or other supplies? There are two things you can do. First, have extra medication and supplies packed in case any unexpected situations arise. Second, ask your physician to write up extra prescriptions to take with you. At least you'll be prepared if you need more. You may also want to ask if you can keep your doctor "on call," contacting him or her in an emergency. If you're going to a foreign country, you may want the prescription translated into the language of that country in case the pharmacist has difficulty understanding English. If you are flying (in a plane!), you should carry medication and other necessary supplies with you. Do not pack all supplies in your luggage. Why? If your luggage ends up in Kansas City when you're flying to Orlando, you don't want to be left without what you need. Besides, if for any reason you need a pill during the flight, it would be rather inconsiderate of you to ask the flight attendant to climb down into the baggage hold to get it!

IDENTIFY YOURSELF!

It's always a good idea to travel with complete identification, not just for your luggage but for yourself. The Medic Alert bracelet, indicating that you have a medical problem, is accepted worldwide as identification of a person with a medical problem. In addition, make sure your wallet contains an identification card with complete details about your condition, the type of medication you need, and any other pertinent information. Again, if you're going to a foreign country, you might make sure that this information is translated into the language of that country. What if foreign languages were never your forte? Try checking with a teacher of that particular foreign language in a local school. Check with the airline that travels to that country. Representatives who speak the language would probably be willing to translate for you. As a last resort, you may want to check with the foreign embassy of that particular country. This may take a little extra time, but your mind will be more at ease when you do travel.

AIRPLANE ANTICS

Let's say your vacation is set, you're flying to Paradise, and you're now making final preparations before leaving for the airport. Any special considerations? You bet!

If you have any physical restrictions, discuss these in advance, either with an airline representative or with your travel agent. Airlines frequently have special services for individuals with restricted mobility. For example, you may be able to board early, select your seat in advance, have wheelchair access to and from the gate, and special meals, if necessary. If you have your own wheelchair and you plan on traveling with it, check with an airline representative to find out what regulations apply.

EATING ABROAD

Foreign eating and drinking occasionally cause problems for any traveler. Therefore, you really have to be on guard against and aware of potential problems. Unless you've been assured that it's o.k., don't drink tap water or even water in thermoses provided by hotels. Avoid fruits or vegetables that may have been washed before being served. Avoid any other foods that include water in their preparation. Even something as simple as brushing your teeth can make you wish you were back home in bed. You've heard of Montezuma's Revenge? Well, Montezuma has traveled to many parts of the world! The best way to conquer the water problem is to use pure, sterilized, or distilled water. Some hotels will provide water purifiers so that you can take water from the tap, process it, and then be able to use it safely.

It is not always safe to even drink typical American soft drinks when abroad. The name of the soft drink may be American, and the packaging may look the same as it does in the United States, but that doesn't mean that it has been made in the U.S. If the drink was manufactured or even bottled locally, you still run some risks. Any foods you do eat should be well cooked and properly prepared. Avoid foods that do not look or smell the way you'd expect them to. It's better to be safe (and hungry) than full and uncomfortable.

If you do want to eat any fruits or veggies, peel them carefully, throw away the peels, and wash them with purified water. If any food has a broken skin or looks damaged, throw it away. You're usually better off not eating any foods that haven't been cooked. Canned baby foods that are available in large markets can be good dietary supplements (remember, you did like them once!) Here is a disappointing thought, however. Pastries, especially those made with cream, can be dangerous (and not just to your waistline!). If they're not taken care of properly, bacteria can grow in them. As far as meats are concerned, be very careful where you eat and what you choose to eat. American laws are very strict about the inspection of meats served to the public. Laws may not be as strict or may even be nonexistent in other countries. Therefore, you run the risk of eating improperly-cooked meats, meats that have not been prepared appropriately, and so on. Use good judgment. You may ask, "Why can't I eat this when the people who live here eat it all the time?" Don't be jealous. You don't know if that's true. You don't know if they eat these foods or if they avoid them, too. Or maybe natives are used to these foods and their lead-lined stomachs can handle foods that your stomach can't. Maybe hundred of natives are home in bed with food poisoning! At any rate, be sure to protect yourself.

Are you beginning to think that, because there is so much to be afraid of, you won't be able to enjoy your vacation? Don't feel that way. Just remember—you're not going on vacation merely to eat. (If you are, don't go someplace where food is such a problem!) Instead, try to emphasize the other, more enjoyable aspects of your trip. Adequate preparation and total awareness are easy to achieve and will certainly help to make your trip an enjoyable one.

CRUISES

More and more cruise ships have special accommodations for people with physical restrictions. Some have rooms specifically designed for individuals with limited mobility. Ramps may be built in and doorways widened. If you're planning on taking a cruise, make sure that you know what ports-of-call the ship will be stopping at. In certain Caribbean ports, for example, the ship does not dock at the pier. Rather, it drops anchor away from the pier and small boats are used to get you ashore. This may be more difficult for you to handle if you have any physical restrictions. Again, if you're taking your own wheelchair, be sure to find out what regulations may apply.

TRAIN TRAVEL

Quite a variety exists in passenger trains throughout the country and abroad. Some trains are very accessible for individuals with disabilities. Others are not as accommodating. If you're thinking of traveling by train, speak with a railroad representative or your travel agent before making a final decision.

BUS TRAVEL

Bus travel is becoming easier for people with disabilities. Even if you need a wheelchair, it can probably be stowed and somebody can help you to get on and off the bus.

A FINAL CONFIRMATION

Remember, not everyone is like Eddie. Many individuals with RA feel absolutely no reluctance to travel anywhere. If you haven't traveled recently, you may want to build up your confidence by taking short trips first. Taking a three-month trip around the world might be a bit much! Even an overnight trip might be traumatic. Start with a couple of day trips, then weekend trips, working your way up to short-distance, week-long excursions. Expanding your travel activities slowly is a good way to develop your confidence. There are special travel agencies for people with disabilities. Look in your local Yellow Pages.

A lot of information has been provided here—mostly precautionary, but nevertheless realistic and sensible. You may need extra time to prepare for your vacation (more time than the "average" traveler). However, with this extra preparation you should be able to enjoy a wonderful vacation, just as anybody else would. Don't forget to send me a postcard!

PART IV.
Interacting With Other People

25

Coping With Others—An Introduction

You do not live your life alone (unless you're reading this book on a deserted island in the Pacific). You interact with many people every day. So you'll certainly want to be able to deal with any difficulties in interpersonal relationships. For example, what are others going to think? How are they going to react? Are they going to ask questions? What kinds of answers will they listen to and what kinds will turn them away? These are some of the questions that may bother you. Since you'll probably be with other people during a good part of your waking hours, it makes sense to be aware of how RA can affect these relationships. Obviously, different problems can exist in different relationships. But before we begin discussing each type of relationship specifically, there are a few general points to be made.

DO UNTO OTHERS . . .

When you interact with others, you don't want to become too wrapped up in your own feelings. If you disregard the feelings of others, you'll also prevent them from getting close to you. Consider how others feel, just as you'd like them to consider your feelings. What does this mean? You're not the only one who has to cope with RA. Important people in your life are also having a hard time, simply because you mean a lot to them. Remember that. Some people tend to feel that their problems don't affect anyone else. You might think, "How can they feel upset? It's happening to *me*!" But is that fair? Take your family, for example. A problem for you is also a problem for them. Of course, it may be affecting you differently. Maybe you're the one experiencing the restrictions, the physical changes, as well as the apprehensions and anxieties, but your condition still affects those who care about you. They don't like to see you suffer. You'll be better able to cope with these important people, as well as help yourself cope better, by remembering this.

YOU CAN'T CHANGE OTHERS

Do you feel that if you try hard enough you can change the attitudes, feelings, or behaviors of others? It doesn't happen that way. Whether they accept your rheumatoid arthritis or deny that you have any problem at all, you can't change them. You can only change yourself. Spend more time working on *you,* and worry less about others. They may change, but it will more likely be a result of the changes they see in you. Help yourself. Be your own best friend.

LOOK THROUGH THE EYES OF OTHERS

If you have an argument with someone, you may believe that you're right and the other person is wrong. In this case, nothing will be resolved. Take a moment and look at the situation through the eyes of the other person. What does he or she see? What might the other point of view be? This will definitely help you to better understand the problem.

If you look at the problem only through your own eyes, someone else's behavior may drive you crazy. Looking through the eyes of others can help you to better understand them and to improve your relationship with them. If you then try to have a discussion, this will also help you to explain how you feel.

PRIDE, YES! REVENGE, NO!

Revenge! There are times when you might think, ''I only wish that _____ could know what it's like to live with RA for an hour, a day, or a week, so that he/she could understand what I've been going through.'' But you know this isn't realistic, and you can't sit around waiting for it to happen. Besides, afterwards you might not be too pleased with yourself for having such vengeful thoughts. So what should you do? Take pride in yourself. Concentrate on doing what's best for *you*. If you have to be a little more self-centered and a little less concerned about what other people think, just accept this as one more way of coping with your condition.

A LITTLE SELFISHNESS IS O.K.

What happens if you're feeling rotten, but others want you to keep doing more and more? In the past, you may have had trouble saying no, because you'd either feel guilty or you didn't want to disappoint someone or hurt their feelings. But now you must curtail your generosity because it can hurt you. Frequently, you may have to give the appearance of being selfish. But don't take this negatively. As long as you don't abuse it, this selfishness can be positive for you. Do for yourself; think of yourself. You're Number One, and that's the way it must be. If you take care of yourself, then you can be in the best shape to deal with others. The reverse does not hold true. If you are best for others, you may not be best for yourself.

BRING ON THE WORLD

Now that we've started with some general ideas, let's see how RA can affect different relationships you may have with people. Of course, not every chapter will apply to you. You can either read the chapters that are appropriate for you, or read them all and realize that different kinds of problems do exist in any relationship.

26

Your Family

Blood is thicker than water! Your family can be a critical factor in your successful adjustment to having RA. Why? You're probably with your family more than with anyone else. If you get along well with members of your family, you'll have a solid foundation from which to move towards a triumphant adjustment to your condition.

There are various types of problems that may pop up with different members of your family. So let's discuss how to cope with each specific member of the family.

COPING WITH YOUR SPOUSE

Of course, having RA has a definite effect on your marriage. But this doesn't mean that problems can't be resolved. Through better communication, understanding, and counseling (if necessary), there are very few problems that can't be worked out. Let's discuss some of the ways in which a marriage may feel the impact of RA.

Social Life Changes

Have you had to cut back on your social activities because of restrictions caused by RA? You may have to curtail some of the activities that you used to enjoy with your spouse. You just may not be able to do as much. This can be hard to bear, especially if you both had active social lives before the onset of your condition. Because your spouse does not have RA, he or she may feel anger, frustration, or helplessness. If, however, your social life is still on hold even after your condition has stabilized, you'll have to ask yourself if this is due to certain fears or apprehensions. If so, refer to other appropriate chapters (such as *Fears and Anxieties*) for suggestions and support.

If Family Responsibilities Must Change . . .

RA may create the need for temporary or permanent changes in each family member's responsibilities. This can surely be another potential source of friction between you and your spouse, especially when your spouse receives a heavy share of the load. "Re-assigning" chores to different members of the family can be very difficult for all.

Stephanie, a 32-year-old mother of two, used to make lunch for her husband and children each morning. But with RA, she was just too stiff early in the morning, and was no longer able to do this. So she "transferred" this responsibility to her husband. Since he had difficulty boiling water, he wasn't too thrilled. He, in turn, placed added responsibilities on the children. This created even more tension. Despite the fact that Stephanie's family loved her and was concerned about her health, they were all understandably upset, especially her husband. How can you change things as smoothly as possible? Make changes gradually. Being able to afford household help would make things easier, of course. But regardless of this, try to avoid overwhelming your spouse. Be realistic in your expectations.

How else can you help your spouse to adjust to greater burdens? Make sure free time is still available for the pleasures of life. It's only when the new responsibilities seem to be all-consuming that serious problems may occur. Look at any changes through the eyes of your spouse. Consider how you'd feel if the situation were reversed. Think how upsetting it would be if you no longer had time for things you enjoyed because of added responsibilities and pressures. Discuss it reasonably, and be gentle.

Denial

What do you do if your spouse simply won't accept the fact that you have RA? You might hear, "Come on, joint pain is no big deal. What are you complaining about?" This is tough to swallow. You can try to "educate" your spouse, but don't go overboard. If you're constantly badgering, reminding your spouse of the things that have changed because of RA, you certainly won't convince someone who has obviously been denying its very existence. Your spouse will not accept your condition until ready to do so. Concentrate on your own feelings. Others' feelings may change, but slowly.

In Sickness and In Health? Sorry!

Unfortunately, some marriages have ended because of chronic illness. The restrictions of RA can drive wedges into what may have previously been good marriages. Former feelings of closeness and intimacy may be replaced by the unwelcome feelings of coldness and distance. Some spouses have so much difficulty accepting changes in appearance and behavior that the "magic" seems to be washed right out of the marriage. But it may not be all your spouse's fault. You may be so apprehensive that you can't enjoy your relationship. Your sensitivity may cause you to be less patient. So marital breakups do occur. But realize that about 50% of all marriages end in divorce anyway, even when RA is not involved!

Statistics aside, what do you do if your spouse is frightened and "wants out?" Your spouse's fear, your own condition, and your fears of abandonment all combine to create a horrible package of anxiety, depression, hopelessness, and panic. This package isn't one you can (or should) handle alone and, at this point, you probably won't be able to talk to your spouse. You may find communication with your spouse either nonexistent or counterproductive. Get some help. Seeking the aid of a professional or an objective outsider may help to smooth over some of the rough edges. If possible, include your mate. But once again, don't force the issue. It's better for you, at least, to get some counseling. If your marriage does end, outside support will be very helpful in getting you back on your feet emotionally.

What About Money?

Rheumatoid arthritis can present added money problems, especially for your spouse. If you are the bread-winner, your spouse may fear the unpleasant role of becoming more responsible for financial aspects of family management. If your spouse is the major income-producer, pressure from the added costs of treatment and medication may be tough. Both you and your spouse will worry about whether all obligations can be met (and continue to be met). Money concerns are frequently a major source of friction in any marriage. Here the problem is just compounded. Sit down, talk it over, and be realistic. Although new strains may arise, these things frequently have a way of working themselves out. Be patient, be communicative, and be positive.

Is Sex Affected?

Another important area in which RA may affect a marital relationship concerns sex. The chapter, *Sex and Rheumatoid Arthritis*, provides more information on this important subject.

A Marital (Con) Summation

Coping with your spouse while you have RA can be extremely difficult and, occasionally, impossible. Any marriage has its ups and downs—its problems that have to be worked out. Having RA makes relationships more vulnerable to crises and arguments. Working through RA-related problems requires much more attention to your spouse's feelings and needs. But it's worth it. If problem spots can be smoothed out, your spouse can really be your best ally in helping you adjust to your condition.

COPING WITH CHILDREN

Children need a lot from their parents. This can surely be frustrating if you're unable to provide as much for them as you'd like. You can't do as much, or help them as much. This does not mean that you don't love them or that you're not a good parent. Because each person lives differently with rheumatoid arthritis, there's no way of predicting how much it will affect you physically (or even emotionally). It may be hard to acknowledge your shortcomings as a parent. But think about your children. How much do they know about your condition? How hard is it for them to deal with? Let's see how you can help them.

How Can I Explain?

The younger the child, the less of an explanation he or she will need. Anything that you tell a youngster will have to be explained simply. Unless you're severely affected, you may not have to say much of anything.

With older children, explanations can be more detailed. Encourage their questions. Timmy, age 9, knew his mother had "a lot of pain in her bones." But his mother couldn't understand why Timmy rarely asked any questions about it. Was he keeping unhappy thoughts inside, or had he just accepted it and didn't feel it was necessary to ask anything? Remember: If your children really don't want to ask you anything, they won't. But let them know that they can if they want to. Upsetting thoughts kept inside can be even more destructive.

The questions of older children will probably be more direct and more specific. Resulting discussions, if handled properly, will not only be helpful for your children—you'll enjoy them! You'll also enjoy the great feeling of closeness that can result.

Fielding Children's Questions

How do you answer questions? This depends on the age of the child, as well as on how much of an answer the child may be looking for. The best advice is to provide direct answers to the specific questions. Don't go into detail, unless your child asks for more information.

Think, for example, about parents talking with their children about sex. Because of the delicate nature of the subject, and the discomfort or anxiety on the part of the parent, more information than necessary is usually given. Have you heard the anecdote about the very young child who walked up to his mother and asked, "Mommy, where did I come from???" The mother started trembling because this was the first time she had heard such a question from her child. But she nervously explained the various parts of the female anatomy and how the sexual act resulted in conception. She told how this ultimately led to the birth of the child. When she finished after about fifteen minutes, she breathed a sigh of relief and expectantly waited for her child's reaction. The child responded, "But Mommy, I didn't want to know all that. I just wanted to know what hospital I was born in!"

The message in this anecdote is clear. Try to determine exactly what your child wants to know. Some children may not even know what answers they are looking for. So just start answering and then ask if that's what they wanted to know. Continue from there.

Be careful not to frighten your child. Children have great imaginations. You don't want your answers to get blown out of proportion. You do want your child to continue to talk to you about your condition. If you show that you accept RA (as much as you can) and the way it affects you, and even welcome questions about it, this will greatly benefit the relationship with your child.

"Will You Die?"

This is an inevitable question. Whenever a child knows that a parent has a serious medical problem, he or she may worry. It may be frightening for your child to see you unable to get out of bed in the morning. You'll have to handle this very carefully. Children become petrified thinking about the death of a parent. They don't understand what you're going through and they will certainly be afraid. Reassure them that you're not going to die. These may seem like empty words, but that's what they need to hear.

Although RA is not considered a fatal disease, it may not be enough for you to tell your child that you will not die, especially if you're not sure yourself. (Children are very perceptive; they'll recognize your fears.) It might be a good idea, therefore, to speak to a professional (your physician or your child's pediatrician, for example) and include him or her in the discussion.

Spending Time

One of the hardest parts of coping with children is handling their disappointment when you can't do all that they'd like you to do. You want to be a good parent. But what does that entail? Most parents believe that they must spend lots of time with their children, taking them places, doing things with them. If this doesn't happen, parents may feel guilty. But RA can be restrictive, and may prevent you from doing a lot of what you'd like to do. You have no choice. How do you solve this dilemma? How do you explain to your child that you can't take him or her somewhere, or that you can't do what you had promised? Children don't want to understand when they're upset. Making deals can help. Explain to your children that you're not available as much as you'd like to be. Come to an agreement with them about some enjoyable activity you can do together when you're feeling better. This arrangement will show your children that you're aware of their unhappiness and want to help.

Try to spend "quality" time with your children—special time when you really share feelings and activities. You shouldn't be as concerned about "quantity" time—the number of minutes or hours you spend with them. If your time together is precious, then this is much more important than the amount of time. Your children will do just fine. Talking with your children and being open with them is another important component in helping them to handle your RA.

COPING WITH ADOLESCENTS

Coping with adolescents can be very different from coping with children. Because adolescents are older and can read more complex material, they can therefore read most of what has been written for adults. They can ask questions if anything they read is too complicated. However, the main difficulty in coping with adolescents is recognizing their unique needs.

The Declaration of Independence

This is the age at which teenagers begin to assert their independence. Look out, world! The future generation is coming! Adolescents want to start moving away from the family setting and its responsibilities. Under normal circumstances, this can create problems in many homes. Your RA can cause even more problems. Why? Because of your condition, your adolescent may have to help out more than usual with daily routines and chores. At the same time, the adolescent wants to do less, and be away more. What a bummer!

For example, 14-year-old Leslie feels guilty about not helping out more at home, but feels that giving in is a sign of weakness (heaven forbid!). This causes Leslie a lot of anguish, which of course she doesn't want to discuss with her parents. The need to escape seems even greater. So, dear parent, imagine how helpful it can be for you to be aware of your adolescent's feelings. Take the initiative and offer a reasonable compromise. Just showing that you understand will help. Maybe things won't seem so hopeless to the adolescent, after all.

The Need for Friends

Adolescents are usually less interested in spending time with family members, and more interested in being with friends. That should make it easier, but it may still be difficult for an adolescent to deal with a parent's RA. Even if the adolescent's friends don't know about your condition, the adolescent may be much more sensitive to the situation. Does this sound strange? Most adolescents want to impress their friends. Somehow, having a parent who has trouble walking doesn't quite "fit the bill." Of course, there are some adolescents who are more mature and open about it. The extent of their love for their parent and a sound family relationship minimize the problem. They may sometimes end relationships with those friends who cannot understand the situation. Unfortunately, however, this is not often the case.

Another problem for your adolescent is transportation (that means you!). Many adolescents count on their parents to drive them to friends' houses, parties, meetings, and so on. But you may not be available (or able) to chauffeur your teenager around as much. As a result, you may feel guilty because you're not being a good parent.

Your teenager, thinking less of you and more of himself or herself, can become upset or even angry. Your teenager may also feel guilty, either because of recognizing this selfishness, or because of feeling like too much of a burden. The best thing to do is to talk it out.

Talking to your Adolescent

Understanding the needs of your adolescent can open the doors to much better communication. However, if you want your talking to be helpful, treat the adolescent like an adult. This will provide the best response. Think about the concerns of your adolescent regarding your condition. Leslie may be very frightened that her mother is never going to get better. However, reassuring her that your condition is fine, and that you're feeling better, may help. If your adolescent feels comfortable talking to you about your RA, encourage it. But remember to respect the rights of those adolescents who would rather not discuss it.

Finally . . .

Your adolescent may shoulder more responsibilities because of your condition. But this may cause problems, especially if your adolescent tries to deny your condition. Some adolescents will be able to deal effectively with their burdens, but some won't. They may simply be unable to handle the pressure. If your adolescent must take on any additional adult responsibilities or jobs because of your condition, consider that he or she may also be ready to enjoy some more adult privileges and pleasures. How can you require teenagers to fulfill adult responsibilities and then restrict them to teenage privileges? If you're apprehensive about their maturity, keep in mind that if they're old enough to do adult chores, they might enjoy some adult privileges as well (within reason, of course). Adolescents will usually be more willing to help out if they know that they will be treated and trusted in a more grown-up way.

COPING WITH PARENTS

Parents have a very hard time dealing with RA, or any illness or condition, in their child (even in an adult "child"). This makes coping harder for you, too. Why? You don't want your parents to suffer or be upset. You'd probably feel guilty about their suffering.

If your relationship with your parents is good, then you're among the lucky ones. But what if you normally have difficulty dealing with your parents? Having rheumatoid arthritis doesn't help! How have your parents treated you since your diagnosis? Do they ignore or minimize your condition? Or do they smother you?

The Ignorers

Janet, a 25-year-old medical assistant living with her parents, began gold treatments for RA less than three months ago. But despite her need for weekly injections, her parents have been showing less and less concern about her condition. They don't ask questions. Even worse, they don't show any interest when she wants to tell them something about it.

Parents who ignore or play down your RA often do this because they can't deal with it. They can't accept the possibility that it might have something to do with them. How? They may be afraid that they did something contributing to the illness or condition. Or maybe they think you inherited the illness or condition from them.

Even if this is far from the truth, it doesn't eliminate the worry underlying such thoughts. To avoid these unpleasant feelings, they may try to deny your having rheumatoid arthritis. They might minimize it, hoping it will all go away.

The Smotherers

Since Fran began her gold injections, her mother has tried to accompany her to the doctor for every appointment. This would almost be understandable, except: 1. Her mother lives fifty-five minutes away by car. 2. Her mother has a heart condition and needs her rest. 3. Fran doesn't want or need company at her appointments. You see, Fran is 34, hasn't lived at home for sixteen years, and often disagrees with her mother's opinions (especially regarding what activities she should participate in and how much rest she should get). Fran certainly feels smothered.

Parents who smother believe that, if you have any kind of problem, they must take care of you. Having rheumatoid arthritis certainly fits this requirement. It doesn't matter what your marital status is, or how old you are. What matters to them is that they are your parents. They are responsible for you and must take care of you. The fact that you can take care of yourself doesn't matter. They'll call frequently, asking how you're doing. They'll want to know what they can do to help. They may come over as often as possible to make sure you're o.k. Whether they come or not, they'll constantly bombard you with questions about your health and activities. What can you do, short of moving out of town and taking on a new identity?

Remember what we said before? It really helps to see a situation through someone else's eyes! Don't you think this holds true here, too? Look at yourself, and your condition, through the eyes of your parents. How do you think they feel? What do they see? You don't have to agree with them, but understanding this will help you talk to them. Looking at your condition through their eyes will also help any discussions you may have with them, as you try to explain how you feel. It's fine to let them know that it bothers you when they do certain things. You'll feel great if your discussions are more productive.

What If Talking Doesn't Help?

If you have tried to talk to them and haven't succeeded, at least you've tried. That will help you feel a little better! At least you won't feel like you should do more—to convince them to switch to your way of thinking! What do you do then? Concentrate more on helping yourself feel better, regardless of whether they understand or not. If they're unhappy with you because you seem to be rejecting their well-meant intentions, so be it.

By the way, if you're unhappy with parents who are ignorers, you'd probably love them to smother you for awhile. And, if you don't like smothering parents, the thought of being left alone is probably very exciting. There's rarely a perfect solution. No one gets along with everyone all the time. Instead of complaining about your parents' faults, try to look at the positives in their behavior. You'll feel better about doing this, too.

How Much Should I Tell?

You know your parents. You know how they react to things. What would you really like to share with them? Would you like to tell them how you're feeling at a particular time? You probably know how they'll react to good news and bad news, and how they deal with unpleasantness. How will you handle their reactions? All these factors will help you to decide how much to tell them.

Sometimes, it's easier to talk with one parent rather than the other. You might tell one parent what's bothering you, and let that parent tell the other. For example, your mother may be able to get through to your father better than you can. This will help everybody.

You might wish you could share unpleasant feelings with a parent because of the reassurance it would bring. It's nice to know that you don't have to face something unpleasant alone. However, what if your parents can't readily accept your problems even if they wanted to? It may be more detrimental for you to tell them things that they can't handle. So don't impulsively tell them anything. Think and analyze. Try to understand what you want to share, and what their reactions may be. It's worth the effort. By spending a little time to figure out what's best, you can help yourself feel a lot better. You'll probably improve your relationship with your parents, as well.

27

Friends and Colleagues

Aside from family, the most important people you'll have to deal with are friends and colleagues. Are there any suggestions for coping with these important people? Of course!

COPING WITH YOUR FRIENDS

What reactions have your friends had about your RA? How many of your friends really know what rheumatoid arthritis is all about? They may have read about it, and at first, they may have thought they knew all about it. But because they weren't physically affected, they might not have been able to really understand what you were experiencing. Some wanted to learn more; some wanted to forget what little they knew.

Some friends may be very supportive—maybe *too* supportive. Other friends may not be supportive enough, something that can bother you even more. Your own mood really determines their reactions. If you don't want them around, if you don't want them close to you, or if you don't want them asking questions and you let them know this, they will probably respect your wishes. But perhaps they won't be there when you really *do* want them around. It's important for you to strike a balance. You may simply want to explain that your feelings change and to please bear with you. You hope they'll understand the fluctuation of your feelings.

Apprehension Keeps Them Away

Friends may not know what to say to you. What should they ask you? How should they talk to you? This can cause so much tension that they don't even want to be with you. They may be so uneasy that they feel, "Why bother?"

Friends may be afraid to call because they don't know how you're feeling. They don't want to run the risk of stirring up unpleasant feelings for you (or for themselves, if they don't know how to respond). On the other hand, there may be times when friends keep asking you how you're feeling and you'd really like to be left alone. Many friendships are lost or hurt because of misunderstandings. These misunderstandings usually involve uncertainty on the part of you or your friends in approaching each other.

Showing Concern

Can anything be done, or are you going to be a hermit for the rest of your life? Don't despair. There are things you can do to improve the situation. Try to set up ground rules with your friends. Tell them how you feel. If you are the kind of person who likes to be asked how you feel, let your friends know. If you'd rather not be asked, let your friends know that, too. If your feelings fluctuate (sometimes feeling talkative about your condition, but at other times reluctant to even think about it), let your friends know. Your changing feelings may be harder for friends to deal with, so let them know that they should talk to you the way they really want to. You'll let them know if and when you're having trouble.

Clear up the question marks. If you tell your friends how you feel and what your needs and desires are, fewer unknowns will exist. The uneasiness about what to do or say, which can hurt friendships, will be reduced. Your friends will become more aware of your needs, and will feel closer to you and less afraid.

Changing Plans

Don't you love having to change plans with a friend because you're so tired that you can't even move? Probably not. So you can understand how your friends might feel if they have restrictions placed on activities. This doesn't have to be so. Good friends, who understand or at least try to understand what you're going through, will probably be able to accept these changes. Others may be less willing to put up with them.

Asking for Help

As you learn to live with RA, do you feel a greater need to call on your friends for help? You may need help cleaning the house, getting places, taking care of children, purchasing groceries, among other things. Are you becoming more selfish? No, but it may seem that way to you. The reality is: There are certain things you must take care of. So if you need help, reach out for it. If your friends complain or show resentment, try to talk it over with them. Don't wait until a friendship is destroyed to realize that built-up problems should have been discussed earlier, when the conflict could have been resolved. If you try and nothing helps, remember this: If your friends still don't understand, what kind of friends are they, anyway?

Asking for Help Appropriately!

If you do need help, figure out who to ask and what they should do. If your friend Myrna loves children, it would probably be better to ask her for help with the kids. If you know that Emma suffers from "supermarketitis," requiring daily therapeutic visits to the local food emporium, then sending her for groceries shouldn't bother her at all. If Mario has a driving phobia, don't ask him to chauffeur you around. Try to arrange for a proper fit when asking for help.

Older, longer-lasting friendships also tend to be stronger and more resilient. Such friends will probably be more receptive if you ask for favors. Newer or more casual friends should probably not be burdened as much. Without giving a friendship a chance to become firmly planted on your hook, you may lose your prized fish— a good, long-lasting friendship. Don't come on too strong. You might think, "But can't they see that I need help?" The answer is, "Not necessarily."

Don't feel like you must do everything yourself. There's nothing wrong with reaching out for help. But you'll feel better if you try to evaluate who to ask for what kind of help. (By the way, when you feel up to it, a nice way to show your appreciation is through an unsolicited gift or gesture.)

Losing Friends

What if it just doesn't work out the way you want? People you thought were your friends don't call or visit. Some are "turned off" by your condition. Maybe they're afraid it's contagious! Others seem reluctant to make any plans with you, saying, "Let's wait and see how you feel." It's sad, but in some cases it just can't be avoided. It's not your decision! You may wonder if it was because the friend couldn't handle your being in so much discomfort. Was your friend uncomfortable about being with you? Was your friend unsure of what to say or do? Whatever the reason, you've probably learned a hard, unpleasant lesson. Although you may feel sad, you can't change someone else's feelings. Be reassured that most people who lose friends because of RA do make new ones. You really don't want a friend who is uncomfortable with you. There may be times, unfortunately, when a friend or lover cannot handle your condition and you may feel like you've been rejected. This can be devastating! You may feel that you have not only been rejected, but you will not be able to develop any other meaningful relationships. This is not true. You are still the same person as you were before, except for the ways that RA has affected you physically. Keep telling yourself that so you can restore any confidence that may have been shaken by this unfortunate rejection.

Usually, however, if rejection occurs or if a relationship breaks up, it couldn't have been too strong to begin with. Many weak relationships have broken up because of medical problems. A sturdy relationship, even if it has to go through some rough times, will probably end up even stronger than before. Remember, you want a friend who likes you the way you are, RA and all! And there are plenty of wonderful, understanding people out there. So don't give up!

COPING WITH COLLEAGUES

We've discussed some of the problems you may have working if you have RA. If you know you're going to work, what kinds of problems might you encounter? You're going to spend several hours each day in contact with the people you work with. You'll certainly want to feel comfortable around them. Let's discuss some ways in which you might encounter difficulties in getting along with your colleagues.

Employer Acceptance or Harassment?

O.k., so you're ready to re-enter the job market. Now you'll worry about whether you should go back to your old job, or whether anyone else would even consider hiring you. What factors come into play? Among them are your prior sickness or absentee record, your present state of health, and the possibility of prolonged absences in the future. The employer will certainly want to consider whether or not you or your medical condition will create any problems on the job. Morale, sick benefits, and liability concerns usually top the list.

The most upsetting cases involve employers who are unwilling to hire you simply because they know about your condition. At this point, you're faced with two choices. You can either give up and look for something else, or you can try to educate the employer (not with your fists!). This can be done through discussions, reading materials, or contact with a physician or nurse. If necessary, your physician can probably reassure your prospective employer that you're fit for the job and should be able to handle it in more or less the same way as someone without RA.

All this groundwork is frequently worth the effort! If you do get the job, your relationship will already be a good one. Greater understanding will exist. In addition, it's nice to know that your employer has at least some insight into your condition.

Now let's look at a different problem. Let's say that you already have your job, but your employer has been expressing his displeasure about curtailed work time. What if an ultimatum is given, stating that if productivity does not improve, you will be discharged (polite, aren't I?)? This is another potential problem. So what do you do? You do the best you can. If an employer doesn't understand enough about RA to know that you must pace yourself, and shows little or no willingness to cooperate, then you're probably better off not continuing employment there. You don't want to look for trouble.

For financial reasons, should you wait until your employment is terminated? This idea has its pros and cons. If you receive unemployment benefits for losing your job, this could ease financial burdens. But if subsequent employers are reluctant to hire you because of the grounds for dismissal, is it worth it? Only you can decide, and you'll probably have to base your decision on your own unique situation. It's a very important question, since your psychological state is so important in your coping with RA. If your employment is aggravating you, then changes may have to be made.

Colleague Conflicts?

There should be little for you to worry about as far as colleagues are concerned. For the most part, if you are comfortable with yourself, others will be, too. Hopefully, colleagues will take it in stride, and won't even think about it. This assumes, of course, that these people *know* about your condition. But what if you don't want to tell anyone? Unless nosy colleagues ask questions, you may decide not to even bother telling them. Obviously, there is no requirement that you do so.

Would it help to provide your colleagues with some basic information on rheumatoid arthritis? It might, although it may not necessarily improve their attitude toward you or the disease. In addition, reading about something doesn't always lead to understanding. However, at least you'll feel better knowing that you've tried to help them understand more about RA. If they don't, they don't. Remember: You can't change somebody else. If a colleague (or anybody else, for that matter) can't handle or understand what's going on, that's his or her problem. You can try to educate people about RA, but don't make it your problem. If you've got an employer with an open mind, that's terrific. Don't be as concerned about other people who don't understand what you're going through. Concentrate more on doing the best *you* can.

Time to Punch Out

Whether you need to work, or enjoy working, you'll certainly want to minimize any potential occupational problems caused by your condition. Take one day at a time. Don't worry about problems that have not, and may never, occur. If your rheumatoid arthritis does cause a problem, be precise in identifying exactly what it is, so that you can employ the best strategies to resolve it.

28

Your
Physician

How do you feel about your physician? (What a question!) Some people see physicians as gods. Others feel that they're rich, unconcerned, cold professionals who don't really want to help. Of course, there are other opinions. What's your feeling? This plays a role in determining how your treatment progresses. You may find that your feelings toward your physician (or physicians in general) have changed since your diagnosis. Some people with RA don't have as much confidence in their physicians, figuring that if their problem had been treated differently, maybe their RA would have been better controlled. It may seem that physicians don't know best, and that you yourself know how you feel better than anyone else. Because of all these feelings, as well as the rising costs of medical care, physicians frequently bear the brunt of much hostility. But physicians *do* want to help.

OFFICE VISITS

Since rheumatoid arthritis can be a serious medical condition, it requires ongoing visits to your physician. These appointments aim to stop any further progression of the disease, and carefully monitor the medication you're taking. Physician visits will also determine if treatment is proceeding properly.

Depending on your condition, the type of treatment you're receiving, and your physician, there may be different types of examinations during the office visit. Different tests are used to check on your health. Blood tests will probably be done at every office visit.

So check-ups are important to keep your condition under control.

Although some patients deny the possibility of any problems and try to avoid regular check-ups, the intelligent person is the one who sees the doctor regularly and as "prescribed."

BEING AFRAID OF YOUR PHYSICIAN

Are you hesitant about speaking to your physician? Perhaps you're afraid of being put in the hospital if your physician finds out how you've been feeling. You might be concerned that your physician will not like the way you're taking care of yourself. You might be afraid your doctor will consider you a complainer who's "crying wolf" and may not listen if an emergency occurs. You might be apprehensive that more aggressive treatment will be necessary, such as unwanted medication or joint replacement surgery. Despite these concerns, you do want your physician to do the best for you. So try to be completely open and honest about the way you're feeling and what you're doing.

STICK UP FOR YOUR RIGHTS

People like to believe that their physicians know what they're talking about. This doesn't mean, however, that you must blindly accept everything that's said. For the most part, physicians respect the patient who asks questions. Disagreement doesn't mean that your physician will throw you out, or even back down. But if you are unsure of why something is being suggested, question it. If you don't like a particular treatment, or it it does not seem to be working for you, speak up. Don't hold back. You do have the right to question. In fact, you have the *obligation* to question. Being unsure is a certain way to be tense. And relaxation is so important. . . .

GETTING SECOND OPINIONS

Because you may not absolutely agree with everything your physician says, and because no physician knows all, you might want a second opinion. You should always get a second opinion before major surgery (unless it's an emergency procedure). But many people are worried about hurting their physician's feelings. Don't let that stop you. Think logically. Most physicians will accept your desire to get a second opinion. It will either confirm what they feel, or will point out the need for further discussion. If your physician objects to your getting a second opinion, you should certainly question why. This *does not* suggest, however, that you should make it a habit of going for second opinions. Nor should you continually shop around for the "ideal" physician. No such person exists.

BEING ABLE TO REACH YOUR PHYSICIAN

Want to get easily frustrated? Try calling your physician for whatever reason (whether it's an emergency or not), and having to wait long hours for your call to be returned. This may be one of your criteria when searching for a physician. Make sure you feel confident in your physician's punctuality in returning your calls.

After you've lived with RA for a while, you'll better learn when you should call and when it's not as necessary. Certain symptoms, such as intense pain, continual stiffness, or high fevers, may require you to immediately contact your physician. Other symptoms, such as minor aches and pains, may not have to be reported immediately. Discuss this with your physician. Find out his or her feelings about your calling if you have problems. Ask about the kinds of things that should be phoned in. Also ask when is the best time to call.

YOU'RE NOT "LOCKED IN"

If you are not happy with your physician, you're not under any obligation to continue seeing him or her. Don't continue a relationship unless it's a good one. Don't continue going to a particular physician if you feel you can't ask questions if you feel intimidated, or if you feel you can't call if there is a problem. Don't stick with your physician if you don't have confidence in what you're told, whether it's about treatment or medication. Finally, don't continue seeing your physician if you feel that he or she doesn't care about you and does not have your best interests at heart.

Your honesty is part of a good professional relationship. If your questions or disagreements hurt the relationship, or if you are afraid of being honest, then this relationship may not be the one for you.

You may want to discuss all of this with your doctor before making any moves. This might straighten things out and improve the relationship. But if it doesn't, remember that you're looking out for your health. You want the support of a physician who can meet most of your needs.

29

Comments From Others

As Ralph Kramden of *The Honeymooners* would say, "Some people have a *B-I-G MOUTH!*" You may agree with this when you think of some of the comments you hear from people around you. They may know you have rheumatoid arthritis, but that doesn't mean they know how to talk to you about it, or what to say. They may say things that they feel are right, witty, intelligent, or even sympathetic. But you may think otherwise! There are times when a certain comment might make you want to implant your knuckles into the speaker's teeth! Or a comment might make you wonder if you're talking to a graduate of the Ignoramus School of Tactlessness.

But why are you reading all this? As you know by now, you cannot change other people. You cannot improve their lack of sensitivity or the way they talk. What you *can* do is learn how to cope with some of the ridiculous comments that you may hear.

ARE OTHERS BEING CRUEL?

Most people really say things out of sincere concern. They may be trying to make you feel better, show their support, or show an interest in you by questioning how you're feeling. Does that mean you must always be receptive to their questions and respond to all of them seriously? It would be nice. The problem is that hearing the same questions over and over can begin to get on your nerves. Initially, you may try to gently respond to comments or questions, or politely change the subject. However, this does not always work. Some people avoid this by simply not telling anyone about their condition. However, if your RA is noticeable, certain comments may be directed toward you anyway.

For the purpose of this chapter, let's assume that we're discussing those comments that you can't avoid, from people who haven't yet learned to tune into your feelings. If you haven't experienced this, that's great! But read on anyway. You never know when what you read might come in handy!

THREE WAYS OF RESPONDING

Many of the things that people say to you may be legitimate comments, but may bug you just the same. Others may not even deserve proper answers. Still others may be said without considering your feelings. But it doesn't matter why the comment is inappropriate. What really matters is how you handle these comments so that *you* feel comfortable. There are three ways that this can be done.

The first way is by ignoring the comments. This is not always easy, especially if the person is waiting for your response, or seems genuinely insulted by your lack of response. How do you get them to stop asking (besides buying a muzzle!)? Change the subject or walk away—ignore the question.

The second way is by trying to answer in a rational and intelligent way, explaining your answer, how you feel, or what you sincerely want to communicate to the other person. But now you may feel like you're banging your head against a wall. What if you just can't convince the other person of what you're trying to say? Such frustration can be painful! There's a limit as to how many times you can try to explain something clearly, and not have it understood or accepted, before you explode. (And this isn't good for your physical health, either!)

What if the first two ways don't do the trick? There's got to be a better way, and there is. The third way is to respond humorously. What does this mean? If someone says something unreasonable to you, or asks you a foolish question that can't really be answered logically, you'll accomplish very little by ignoring it or trying to reasonably explain your feelings. You don't know if your answer will be accepted or if the interrogation will continue. So, in many cases, the third option may be best. This is called "paradoxical intention." The idea behind it is that the person is asking or saying something that is really unanswerable. So you're going to have a little fun with your response. Let's see how it works.

HANDLING THE "BIG MOUTH" SYNDROME

What might you hear? And how should you handle it? Remember, the best response is one that will educate the "commenter." You'd like to explain your situation nicely, in a non-offensive, sincere way. But you're only human. So how can you respond when you get fed up? Read on . . .

"You Look Awful!"

It can be very upsetting when somebody says, "Wow, you look lousy!" You may feel lousy but you certainly don't want to be reminded of it. You surely don't want to think that the way you feel is so obvious to others. You'd like to at least believe that you look o.k. to those around you. Even if it's said sympathetically, being told that you don't look well may be insulting. So what do you say? You might respond, "Thank you, so do you!" Or, "Yes, I know. I've worked hard to look that way." Or if you're really in a cynical mood, you might say, "I know I look lousy. That comes from hearing people tell me this!" Of course, you could always say, "That makes sense, since I don't feel so hot, either!"

"Why Do Your Fingers Look Like That?"

Most considerate people won't ask ridiculous questions such as this. But every now and then, you might encounter someone who is so absorbed with himself or herself that common courtesy is overlooked and curiosity takes over. So what do you do if you don't want to explain how the inflammation of RA has affected your joints? You might say, "My fingers did too much walking through the Yellow Pages." Or "That's what happens when you strangle people who ask questions like that!" Of course, you could put the other person on the spot by asking, "What's wrong with them???" as you smile innocently!

"What Are Those Bumps On Your Arms?"

Few people are tactless enough to ask questions like this, unless they've really never heard of rheumatoid nodules. But even then, this isn't the brightest of questions. So how should you respond? How about, "My real name is Pinocchio, but it isn't my nose that grows." Or, "I was beaten by four pregnant gorillas and the swelling still hasn't gone down!"

Remember: For this approach to work best, you want to respond in a light-hearted way. This will show the person making the comment that you're fine, but you just don't appreciate what he or she is saying.

"Are You Sure You Needed Joint Replacement Surgery!"

What if a friend finds out that you've had a hip replaced and says, "You should have gotten a second opinion. You probably don't need it." Besides retorting that you *did* get a second opinion, how else can you respond to this? You might answer by saying, "You're right—I don't need it. I just love being confined to bed!" Or else, "You're right—I should have gone to more doctors. The smell of the antiseptic waiting room excites me!" Or, "I decided that I needed it so my leg would be strong enough to kick you in the *#@''#''!"

"What Did You Do To Yourself?"

Some people are convinced that, whenever something goes wrong, it is a result of personal neglect. You meet a friend in the street who says, "If only you had eaten better, this wouldn't have happened." You could reply, "What should I eat now, a new joint?" Or, "If you want to see what great shape I'm in, sit back while I clobber you!" If someone asks why you seem tired, you might respond, "Normally I don't seem so tired, but I just finished a marathon dance contest." Or you could say, "I'm tired from kicking people who keep asking me what I did to myself!" This does not suggest that you be unfeeling in your answers. However, if you need to let the "commenter" know that you don't appreciate these questions, that'll do it!

"How Can You Stand So Much Pain?"

In response to this profoundly sympathetic expression of curiosity, you might want to ask, "What pain? The pain from my joints or the pain I get from these dumb questions!" Or you might want to point out other feelings, such as, "I've grown rather accustomed to not being able to move!" Or you might simply say, "I don't stand it. I usually have to lie down!" People will get the message. You may not like the pain of RA, but at least you're learning to cope with it.

"What's Rheumatoid Arthritis?"

Plenty of people are aware of what arthritis is, even if they don't know specifically about rheumatoid arthritis. But how do you respond if somebody asks what it is, or says, "I never heard of RA," and you're tired of explaining? You might say, "Let's forget you even brought it up. Then you can keep your streak going!" Or you could say, "I never heard of it either. How's the weather?" Don't forget: You really don't want to hurt the person's feelings by being sarcastic. However, coping with comments from others can be one of the hardest things about living with RA. There are times when being gentle and tactful with others is less important than helping yourself to handle comments without becoming aggravated.

If the person asks why you sound sarcastic, you can explain that you're not trying to be that way. But the comment you just heard was so ridiculous that you figured the person was trying to be funny. So you decided to have some fun, too! But if the person really wants to know how you feel . . .

You won't always have to use this technique, but you may want to. You'll always come across someone who will say or ask something ridiculous. However, as you learn to feel better in your responses to comments, you'll find that you can handle them more calmly. You won't have to use sarcastic-type comments, and you'll have more fun with humorous, enjoyable ones. You'll keep people on your "friend" list, rather than on your "you know what" list.

What if you're thinking, "I could *never* say those things. It's just not my style." Well, you don't always have to. But you can at least *think* these comments. Even that will help you to feel better!

OTHER LOVABLE COMMENTS

What are some of the other comments that you may hear? How many of these have come your way—"Is rheumatoid arthritis contagious? . . . How do you get dressed? . . . Why don't you quit your job? . . . You should exercise more! . . . Are you sure you can walk up those stairs? . . . Your hands look strange! . . . Rest. Don't do anything . . . What did the doctor say? . . . How's your hip? . . . What is the prognosis? . . . Wow, have you changed! . . . You must miss the way it was . . . What's the matter with you? . . . Can I help you? . . . I certainly don't envy you . . . Your having rheumatoid arthritis is the worst thing I ever heard!"

IS THAT ALL?

It would fill volumes to include all of the comments that you might hear from well-meaning friends or relatives. By reading these examples, you can at least get an idea of how to respond in a humorous way. Look over this list. Can you come up with some goodies? You don't want to be cynical or cruel. Rather, you want to show the speaker that you're feeling well enough to respond light-heartedly.

A FINAL COMMENT

One of the most common and yet most irritating comments that you may hear has been saved for last. Imagine somebody who is supposedly sympathetic, and trying to help you feel better, turning to you with eyes full of compassion and concern, saying, "I heard about someone who was crippled from rheumatoid arthritis!" As you turn to walk away, you respond, "I heard about someone who was crippled after telling someone with RA what you just told me!" You walk away, head held high and a smile on your face, leaving the astonished well-wisher behind you.

30

Sex and Rheumatoid Arthritis

This chapter is *not* rated R, for Restricted. Rather, it is rated E, for Essential. Why? If you are sexually active, living with rheumatoid arthritis can certainly have an impact on your sex life.

Has RA decreased your sexual appetite or ability? This can have an important bearing on the closeness of the relationship with your partner. What kind of sexual relationship did you have before you were diagnosed? (I'm not being nosy. You don't have to write and tell me!) Was it a solid one, or was it on shaky ground? If you had a good sexual relationship, you'll have an easier time getting over any obstacles that RA may have thrown into your sex life. If your sexual relationship wasn't good, it is unlikely that having RA will make it better. You may need some professional help to keep things from breaking down altogether. But all hope is not lost. If you unite with your partner to work things out together, reassuring each other, re-learning how to please each other, showing a desire for each other, progress can certainly be made.

WHERE'S THE PROBLEM?

Let's talk about what the problems might be. There can be both physiological and psychological reasons for changes in your sexual appetite. Physiological problems are better suited to specific treatments. Psychological problems are harder to deal with (ah, there's the rub). Let's explore some of the different possibilities.

The Body Beautiful? (Physical Problems)

Can physical problems alter your interest in sex? You bet your hormones they can!

There is no question that RA can have an effect on your sexual life. What can cause some of the difficulties? How about pain, stiffness, and fatigue? Most sexual problems are related to pain and joint restrictions, since the genitals are not really specifically affected by arthritic problems.

It's very hard to enjoy sexual activities or even engage in them at all if you're in a lot of pain, or if sex itself becomes painful. If RA affects larger joints, such as the hip, elbow, or knee, sex may certainly be affected.

Because painful movement or restriction of joints can make sex difficult, it's important to explore possible ways of changing this. Try procedures that can help relax your muscles or reduce pain, such as moist heat, warm baths, or compresses. Limbering-up exercises may pave the way to more pleasurable sexual encounters. (This gives new meaning to the phrase ''warm-up,'' doesn't it?)

Since sexual activity often takes place at night, aspirin (or other pain-killing medication) may be taken before the sexual act so that pain relief is at its maximum.

You may want to try different positions. Some of them may put less of a strain on painful or restricted joints. If sexual activity is painful, you may be better off taking a more passive role in your encounters. Assume a less active position. On occasion, the use of simple devices such as pillows or knee pads can make sex a lot less painful.

Is there any particular time of day when you experience less pain? For some people, it may be too uncomfortable to have sex late at night. Others may be too stiff in the morning or the early part of the day. Working these problems out takes the cooperation of both partners. Kids, work, or other responsibilities may interfere, of course, but it's better to have sex at planned times than not at all. Frequently, sexual problems can be helped by using your imagination and experimenting with different varieties (in position, timing, and techniques).

Other physical problems can affect either men or women. For example, fatigue can be a factor. If you're tired, you're going to be less interested in sexual activity. This can be a real headache! (Sorry about that!) But if you're uncomfortable or fatigued, hanky-panky will just have to be put on hold. Is this a poor choice of words?

Actually, it may be an excellent idea. After all, just holding each other can be a wonderful experience, too!

What about drugs? Sexual problems may be caused by such medication as painkillers, sedatives, and tranquilizers, or by other types of "drugs" like alcohol. It's true that small amounts of any of these may make you feel more relaxed (increasing the possibility of sex), but too much can work against you. The use of alcohol is notorious in reducing sexual abilities because of its effect on the body.

Some drugs can have a direct effect on sexual desire. For example, certain medication (such as tranquilizers, which reduce your anxiety) can suppress sexual desire or your ability to achieve orgasm. Antihypertensive medication may also have an effect on sexual performance.

Some women may experience vaginal dryness. This can be a problem, since dryness can make intercourse so painful that you'll want to avoid it. (It may also cause bleeding.) But think of vaginal dryness as a lack of excitation. Dryness is not an unusual complication of RA. If dryness causes painful intercourse, what can you do? Keep in mind that a longer period of foreplay can increase vaginal lubrication. Otherwise, consider using water-soluble lubricants such as KY jelly. This can ease the dryness that might otherwise interfere with, or prevent, sexual activity.

What about sex after joint replacement (or other) surgery? Sexual relationships can, in many cases, be resumed once healing has taken place. But make sure you consult your surgeon before resuming sexual activity.

The return to sex can be either extremely pleasurable or extremely disappointing, depending on each participant's point of view. If you were looking for skyrockets, but were very nervous, maybe you were disappointed. Inability to perform is not unusual following surgery, hospitalization, or painful flares, because of fears that sexual exertion may worsen the situation. But that doesn't mean it's always going to be this way. Once some of your concerns have been alleviated, you can be more spontaneous. This can bring about lots of pleasure.

Going Out of Your Head? (Psychological Problems)

Your body isn't the only thing that may affect your sexual interest. Your mind also comes into the picture.

What's the most important sex organ? Think hard now. The correct response is: your brain! (Did I catch you?) If a sexual problem exists that is not physiological, then it doesn't exist in your body, but in your mind.

Many people with RA experience a decreased interest in sex. This doesn't necessarily mean there's something wrong with you. As a matter of fact, decreased sexual interest is common in many chronic illnesses.

Self (and Body) Image

Living with RA may affect your self-esteem. Do you like yourself less because of your condition? If you feel this way, you may be more fearful of rejection by your partner. As a result, you may reduce sexual activity simply to minimize the chances of rejection.

Because self-esteem is a necessary factor in enjoying sexual intimacy, you'll want to improve your ability to like yourself. Feeling good about yourself and your body are very important if you want to enjoy your sexual relationships. It will also make your partner feel more comfortable. On the other hand, if you don't feel good about yourself, this will also affect your partner. This can certainly interfere with closeness!

Related to low self-esteem is an altered body image. Loss of satisfaction with your own body can decrease your self-esteem. You may feel reluctant to share your body with your spouse or partner. Do you see your body in a distorted way? Alice, a 47-year-old woman married for twenty years, was upset that her condition had resulted in a few joint deformities. She feared that her husband would not want her to touch him because of the way her hands looked. Do you fear that your partner may be less interested in sex because of the way you look? Actually, your partner may not feel this way. But you may try to avoid it anyway, rather than risk rejection.

Self-consciousness can be a big problem. Some people with RA feel less feminine or masculine because of changes in the way they move or look. How has your condition affected your perception of your sexuality? If having RA makes you feel less of a person sexually (and interestingly, this is not uncommon), then you've targeted an important area to work on. See what things you can change (consider getting advice about clothes, make-up, and other "appearance enhancers"). Try to remember that nobody's perfect. Everybody has flaws. It makes sense to work on enhancing your looks in whatever ways are appropriate. If you are overweight, wear fashions that will trim down your appearance. If you have a big nose, apply make-up so as to give the illusion of a slimmer one. Whatever the problem, there is usually a way to correct it. But improving your mental attitude is just as important. For those problems that can't be modified, use some of the thought-changing procedures described earlier in this book. They may be the key to your future happiness!

Emotional Interference

Emotions can get in the way, too! Sexual activity may be restricted because of depression. You may be so withdrawn that you simply have no interest in it. Anxiety concerning sex itself, the intimacy of your relationship, or performance, can also hold you back. You may be afraid that you just can't "make it."

Any of these things can happen in any situation—not just with RA. Fortunately, they can also be changed with proper awareness, interaction, improved communication, and therapy (if necessary).

Maybe you're afraid of getting pregnant. Even if you use a contraceptive, you may still be nervous, and this may make it hard for you to enjoy sex spontaneously. But sex does not have to be spontaneous in order to be pleasurable. And perhaps there are additional things you can do to decrease your chances of pregnancy. Discuss this with your physician before moving into separate bedrooms!

Sexual problems can be frustrating, especially if you don't have a partner. It may be uncomfortable for you to even think about finding someone now, knowing the problems you're having with RA. Take things one step at a time. Be more social, look to make new friends, and try not to worry about the more intimate activities which might occur in the future.

TALK IT OVER

A very important part of sexual relationships is communication. If you and your partner can share thoughts and feelings, you'll be in much better shape to work out any sexual problems that may occur as a result of your condition. If communication problems exist, however, difficulties may be very hard to resolve.

It is important to discuss sexual problems with your partner. Ruth, a 38-year-old housewife, had RA. Her husband Bill felt incapable as a lover because (1) He was unable to get Ruth excited, and (2) He caused her pain whenever he attempted to make love to her. But Bill may be reassured to know that these problems could be a result of RA rather than his inadequacy as a lover. If that's the case, then both Ruth and Bill should explore different methods of igniting sexual fires. Otherwise, unpleasant feelings may develop between them. You can work through such feelings, however. Acknowledge the problem and discuss it with your partner. It can be very helpful to discuss any problems with your physician or other health professional as well. In many cases, the major problem is that you keep these feelings inside, avoid discussing them, and cause your sexual life to dwindle down to nothing.

Try to maintain nice, wide-open lines of communication with your partner. Discuss any sexual problems openly. You may even want to discuss them with your physician or another professional, to determine whether they are physiological or psychological. You'll then be better able to work on them.

All that has been said, of course, assumes that your interest in sex is affected by your condition, and that your partner is suffering. But what if the opposite is true? What if you still have normal sexual desires, but your partner is the one who's afraid? Maybe there's a fear of hurting you, or creating additional problems. Or maybe you're regarded as a fragile flower, easily broken, and your partner is reluctant to be sexually spontaneous. This must be carefully discussed. If one-on-one attempts at working things out don't help, don't hesitate to get some professional assistance. It's well worth it.

AND NOW THE CLIMAX

Because sex is such an intimate and important part of a marriage (or any serious relationship), the whole relationship can be affected when either or both partners feel there is trouble. Try to discuss this. If necessary, include your physician in a discussion to clarify issues that may not be as readily accepted. You can still have a warm relationship even if your sex life is less active, but not if there are bitter feelings and misgivings at the same time. Understanding each other's feelings is a very important part of coping with RA.

Remember: Having RA doesn't mean that sexual activity must be reduced, curtailed, or totally eliminated! As a matter of fact, it can still be as pleasurable and as important as the partners want it to be. (By the way, as long as we're talking about the climax, are you aware that orgasm triggers a release of naturally-produced pain-killers? What an effective way to reduce pain in a pleasurable way!)

31

Pregnancy

To have a baby, or not to have a baby. That is the conception. Whether it is nobler (or safer) to have children may be a big question mark. Why? You may be afraid that rheumatoid arthritis may cause a difficult or unsafe pregnancy. You may be concerned that your children will "catch" RA. Let's consider some of the important issues regarding pregnancy.

DOES PREGNANCY AFFECT YOUR RA?

Pregnancy can place additional stress on you, although it is impossible to predict what will happen during anyone's pregnancy. It's possible that you'll feel better than usual during your pregnancy. It's interesting that, in some cases, symptoms of rheumatoid arthritis are even relieved during pregnancy. But don't get used to this. They'll probably return once the pregnancy is over. Other than this, pregnancy shouldn't have any major long-range effects on your RA, either beneficial or harmful. As a result, you'll probably decide to attempt (or avoid) pregnancy for the same reasons that others would under non-RA circumstances.

DOES RA AFFECT YOUR PREGNANCY?

Unfortunately, your pregnancy may not be event-free if you have RA. Individuals with RA have a statistically greater chance of premature births and neonatal complications. There is a greater chance of miscarriage, and there is a small possibility of congenital abnormalities.

Other problems may affect you, the mother, because of RA. For example, if your condition has affected rib joints, it's possible that pregnancy may be uncomfortable or difficult. This could be because it's more difficult to breathe abdominally. If your hips have been affected, it may be difficult for delivery to take place. If your legs cannot be properly positioned, a Cesarean section may be necessary. If your lungs have been affected, you may experience a little more shortness of breath.

Besides these, other problems that can disrupt any normal pregnancy can still occur. Such pleasures as morning sickness, nausea, and fatigue are still possible. Thrilling, right?

CONCEIVING

Will you have more difficulty conceiving because of RA? Probably not, although some women have problems conceiving regardless of their medical condition. There is some evidence that women with RA may be somewhat less fertile than others. However, it's not exactly understood why this is so.

When you and your spouse decide to try to have children, check with your physician to make sure there are no other reasons why you should hold off. For example, it's probably not a good idea to attempt to conceive while you're in the middle of an RA flare. This doesn't mean that you can't try, however, or that something will go wrong if you conceive while in a flare. But you'll probably want your condition to stabilize so you'll be in the best possible shape for your pregnancy if it does happen. Speak to your doctor. Each case should be discussed individually. (In addition, you might not want to consider expanding your family if you're having difficulty fulfilling all of your current responsibilities.)

Are you concerned that there may be a possible genetic factor involved in RA? You may be concerned about passing rheumatoid arthritis on to your children. Although there are definitely families in which several members have RA, most cases of RA do not seem to be inherited. It has never been clearly proven that RA is transmitted genetically. At best (or at worst?) there are some who believe that a person may be born with a susceptibility to RA, but that it still takes something to trigger off or develop the disease. So relax.

IF YOU DO CONCEIVE

If you do become pregnant, it is essential to remain in close contact with your doctor. This is especially important because you have a chronic medical problem. This way, if any problems do develop, you'll be able to "nip them in the bud."

Although you may have had an obstetrician before you were diagnosed with RA, be sure that he or she will take care of you now, considering your medical condition. Some may prefer not to treat individuals with RA and will suggest switching to a different obstetrician. Is this wrong? You may not be happy about it, but you certainly want to know if a physician feels uncomfortable.

MEDICATION AND PREGNANCY

In general, it's usually a good idea to avoid most medication during pregnancy. But this is not always possible. Aspirin, for example, has been used by many women during their pregnancies, without any damage to the fetus. Other medication, such as gold or prednisone, has been used during pregnancy (although if it can be avoided, do so). It's probably not a good idea to begin treatment with powerful drugs (such as gold) during pregnancy.

There is certain medication which shouldn't even be considered during pregnancy, such as the immunosuppressive drugs. If you're on any of these, don't even attempt to conceive yet. Wait for your doctor's go-ahead after discontinuing their use.

In all cases, don't take decisions regarding medication and pregnancy lightly. And, even more importantly, don't take decisions into your own hands. That's what you have a doctor for, right?

What if you discover that you're pregnant while you're on medication? Your doctor may want you to stop the medication as soon as possible. It's o.k. to stop some medicines abruptly. But remember that it is possible that you'll experience a flare-up from discontinuing their use.

Whether or not you should continue medication, stop it, or even consider pregnancy is a matter that you'll want to discuss with your family and your doctors (not just your rheumatologist, but your obstetrician and maybe even someone involved in high-risk pregnancies).

ARE YOU PACIFIED?

As you can see, there are plenty of question marks. Should you become pregnant? What about your medication? What about selfishness or guilt feelings? Will you really be able to care for the baby if your RA is so bad that you can't hold him, diaper him, or feed him?

What about breastfeeding? Will your medication enter the breastmilk and, in turn, the baby?

The best thing to do is to bring all issues out into the open and discuss them—husband and wife, doctor and family, obstetrician and rheumatologist. Everyone must get involved in the discussion. We're not dealing with simple questions such as "Should I take two aspirin today or one?"! We're talking about major considerations which have significant psychological overtones, too.

Remember: In most cases, pregnancy should not be a problem at all, especially if you have only a mild case of RA. What's the key to a successful pregnancy? Awareness, supervision, and careful planning. Take all these factors into consideration, and then—good luck!

PART V.
Living With Someone With Rheumatoid Arthritis

32

Living With Someone With Rheumatoid Arthritis—An Introduction

Illness can create changes in relationships. No kidding! If you live with someone who has RA, you may have a number of concerns. You may now see that person differently. Maybe you are reminded of your own vulnerability. Maybe you were dependent on that person before—now you have to shoulder more of the burden. What does all this mean? Although you share the concerns of the individual who has rheumatoid arthritis, you also worry about yourself. If you have difficulty dealing with your loved one because of RA, you're not alone. Often, illness in a loved one creates a lot of ambivalent feelings in yourself. Concerns about the future, your loved one's health, and money may be troublesome to you. This is not unusual.

What if you feel anger towards this person, not because of anything that was done, but because of the fact that RA has created changes? This is normal, but may still produce guilt. Why? Because this anger is directed towards somebody who, at the present time, is vulnerable and unable to defend himself or herself. (By the way, throughout this book I have purposely avoided calling the person with RA a "patient," simply because I believe in emphasizing the *person* rather than the *condition*. However, for the sake of convenience and because repeating "your loved one" can become tedious, in these last few chapters I will refer to the person with rheumatoid arthritis as the patient.)

WHAT CAN YOU DO?

If you are close to someone with RA, you have an important job on your hands.. This job is made up of many components, the most important of which is the need to be understanding and supportive. This is very important, whether you live in the same house as the patient or are simply a relative or friend. Remember: People with RA do not have it easy, but they'll have a much harder time if they feel alone and isolated.

LOYAL LEARNING

A great way for you to help is by learning as much as you possibly can about rheumatoid arthritis and its treatment. Do you enjoy worrying? You may have unnecessary worries if you don't know things about RA treatment that the patient does. By understanding the patient's program, you can better provide support and understanding.

LOYAL FOLLOWING, OR LETTING GO

Don't stay on top of the patient. Sure you'll want to help. But give the patient enough space to regain some control over his or her own life.

How about doctor's visits? If the patient agrees, you may want to go along for the ride. There may be times when the doctor might want to discuss something with you. It might be a good idea for four ears rather than two ears to listen when the doctor is explaining RA, medication, or other aspects of the treatment program. However, if the patient wants to go alone, and feels strongly about it, don't force the issue.

ENCOURAGE, DON'T PESTER

Encourage adherence to proper management routines or medication needs. But don't badger. If the patient is not taking proper care of himself or herself, there is a limit as to how much you can do to change things. Screaming usually doesn't help (and it can hurt your vocal cords!). Should you tell the physician if the patient is not taking care of himself or herself? That's a hard question to answer. You don't want to overstep your bounds and be resented. At the same time, you don't want to sit back and let the patient create unnecessary problems. This is especially true if the patient doesn't seem to care. What do you do if the patient just "gives up?" Play each situation by ear. In deciding whether or not to say anything, you should discuss it first with the patient. Voice your concerns, mention that you're afraid of a problem becoming worse. Listen to the responses before deciding whether to carry it any further.

SYMPATHY?

Because of the difficulties of living with RA and its treatment, you may sympathize with the patient. You may feel sad about what he or she has to go through. This may help you to provide beneficial support. But don't pity the patient. This can be destructive.

There will be times when the patient is so fatigued that little or nothing can be done. At such times, it is not appropriate for you to insist that the person "get up and do something." That won't make him or her feel better! Try to help out. Try to reduce the patient's pressures at that time. See if you can take over any of his or her obligations or responsibilities; this will certainly make things easier.

At the same time, don't allow the patient to baby himself or herself. In general, if the patient can do something (even if it takes time), let the person do it. If you feel that the patient is "copping out" or malingering, this is something you should both discuss. Try to make life as normal as possible for the patient.

DON'T BE EXTREME

Frequently, friends or relatives go from one extreme to the other. What does this mean? When the patient gets tired, you'll help out. But when the person is no longer tired, will you allow him or her to do what is desired? When feeling better and able to do things, the last thing the patient wants is to be told to get into bed and rest. Have faith in your special someone. If the patient really doesn't feel well, he or she will rest. Otherwise, let 'em be!

HOW TO RESPOND

Can you always be sure of the best response to the patient? You may feel that, at certain times, the best way to respond is with sympathy and understanding. At other times, the best thing may be to just ignore what's going on and walk away. There may be times when you want to joke about RA. But there's no way for you to know for sure. You can't predict the needs of the patient. How to help? Lay ground rules. Hopefully, the patient will initiate this. If not, maybe you can start the discussion. Mention your concerns. Talk about your interest in being as helpful as you possibly can, and ask what you can do to help. Things will move more smoothly if you have a good idea of what to do and when to do it. Even if there are no clear-cut, definite answers, at least there will be some constructive communication. You'll be better able to handle future problems.

KEEP TALKING

It is very important to have open lines of communication between you and the patient. This is the only way you can really hear how he or she feels, both physically and emotionally. In this way, you can truly be of help. This doesn't mean that the conversations will always be pleasant. Talking about problems, depression, fears, or joint pain isn't very enjoyable, especially if you don't have any answers. But with good communication, any difficulties will be overshadowed by the feeling of closeness resulting from shared feelings and concerns.

The majority of this book has been directed toward the person with rheumatoid arthritis. These chapters, however, are designed more for the non-RA person. This information can help you to see the patient's unique experiences through his or her own eyes. The next two chapters will help you to understand more about what children and adolescents with RA may go through.

33

The Child With Rheumatoid Arthritis

If a child is diagnosed as having JRA, it is very likely that his or her doctor will immediately have two or three new patients: the child, and the child's mother and/or father. This may be only the tip of the iceberg. The diagnosis of a child with any serious problem can have a devastating effect on the child's family. It's important for family members to work through any emotional difficulties they may experience as a result of a child's JRA. This will keep the family intact and will help the child to cope with his or her condition. Who else is involved? Friends, teachers, other relatives—all can be affected.

THE CHILD'S PARENTS

The parents of the child will probably experience a whole range of emotional reactions. Feelings of guilt and intense anguish are not uncommon. They may feel that they have genetically transmitted the problem to their child, although this is unlikely. Perhaps they did not use the right physicians, or didn't take proper care of the child. "Is there something we could have done to prevent this?" parents may exclaim. All these thoughts are usually emotional, but can be destructive unless they are worked through. Parents should not attempt to communicate these feelings to the child. Nor should parents make the child feel ashamed.

Watching your child experience pain as he tries to move can be horrible. It's also hard for the parents to make sure that the child takes all necessary medication, and follows the proper treatment program, such as exercising regularly or getting enough rest.

HOW TO TREAT THE CHILD

You don't want to make things harder for the child with JRA. So don't behave any differently from the way you always did. Don't be more harsh and disciplining, or more lax and indulging. If you would really rather help the child adjust, then treat the child as a child, not as an unfortunate youngster with JRA. Parents: Avoid changes in the way you raise your child.

Try not to show painful or unhappy reactions to the child. Imagine how the child will feel seeing unhappiness in loved ones. You can be sure the child will feel guilty. This will only make things worse.

Brothers and sisters at home will definitely be affected. The degree to which siblings are affected varies, however. This depends on how much extra attention the child with JRA receives, and how brothers and sisters react to this extra attention. Do the other siblings feel like they're losing time with you or other relatives? They may feel that they're being "pushed aside" because of the sick sibling. This can cause tension between the child with JRA and your other children. Brothers and sisters may become resentful of the extra attention given to the ill sibling. They may not believe that JRA is such a big deal, but think that it is being blown out of proportion for extra attention. On the other hand, the child with JRA may not even want all this attention. This can create guilt!

A CHILD WITH JRA, NOT A JRA CHILD!

Emphasize the *child* rather than the *condition*. It is better to think of or talk about your child as still a child—a child who happens to have JRA. In addition, try to maintain a calm, emotionally-stable home. This is crucial to keep the family together. It is harder to change the behavior of more distant family members. How can you keep telling friends and relatives not to bring gifts or shower extra attention on your "poor child?"

As we've said before, parents (as well as others who are close to the child) should learn as much as possible about JRA. The more knowledge you have, the more understanding you can be. You can then be more supportive of your child.

THE CHILD CAN HELP HIMSELF OR HERSELF, TOO

Managing your child's RA should be done matter-of-factly. Make it a regular part of life. It's usually not a good idea to give rewards to your child just for following normal JRA treatment routines. You want the child to learn proper self-care habits, not to expect a reward.

Regular family habits should continue as before. You all have to learn to live with any restrictions that JRA may impose. Hopefully, everyone in the family, especially the ill child, will feel more at ease with your child's primary physician. In that way, any questions or concerns can be dealt with. Your child, especially if very young, will be less able to understand the facts about JRA. The child may ask, "Why do I have to go through all this?...Why do I have to take all these pills?...Why do I always hurt so much?" Other questions may also occur. You want your child to be able to ask questions, even if you can't provide all of the answers.

HOW DO CHILDREN COPE?

An important factor in determining how well a child will adjust to JRA and its treatment is how well the child handled stress *before* the onset of the condition. (Does this sound familiar? Of course. This also helps you to understand how adults adjust!) But having JRA is very difficult for a child, especially if growth problems result, and if physical restrictions interfere with normal activities. You'll want to do everything you can to help the child deal with this. Other problems that may occur for adults can also plague children, such as feelings of isolation, pain, unhappiness with body image, and the side effects of medication. So what do children do? Some withdraw, sleeping as much as they can, staying away from friends (and even family), and keeping their bodies covered at all times. Others are very open about their condition. They almost flaunt it, trying to get extra attention. But most children with JRA fall somewhere between these two extremes. Coping strategies are sometimes used, however, which you may recognize as a sign of unhappiness.

Children Deny, Too!

Children may try to deny some aspects of having JRA. They may not concentrate on proper exercise or maintenance routines, and may "forget" about their pills. They may want to do all the things they used to do. So children may deny that they have a problem. But if they push it away, does that mean it doesn't exist?

You want your child to do what's best. But there are times when children may be able to do more than you think they can. In many cases, children are less sensitive to pain and other negative aspects of the illness than adults. Often, *you* may be more concerned about the JRA than your child! Try not to be overprotective. However, you should still protect your child. Even when your child pushes too hard, try to allow the child to learn for himself or herself what can and cannot be done. In order to mature while having JRA, the child must be aware of any limitations that may exist.

"Lashing Out"

Rebellion against authority is a normal part of a child's development. When it happens, be sure that you are ready and prepared to deal with it. At the same time, be assured that a child with JRA will probably not seriously hurt himself or herself with tantrum behavior. So deal with rebellion the same way you would if your child didn't have JRA. Ignore it, wait until the child has calmed down, and then talk to your child. Do try to minimize the physical effects of these outbursts. Try to keep the home environment emotionally calm, stable, supportive, and loving.

On the Positive Side

Children like to participate in the same sports that their friends do. However, soccer may not be the best sport for hip, knee, or foot problems; volleyball may not be good for hand or wrist problems. Still, many children want to play with their friends so they won't be seen as "outsiders." If your doctor approves, it may be o.k. to let the child try to participate, but if flares occur, or the doctor determines worsening or more damage to the joints, then *stop*.

Some children can be encouraged to learn other enjoyable activities. Swimming is a great sport, and is good for RA. Why not encourage that? Other non-physical activities, such as chess, or arts and crafts, can be good outlets. And, of course, doing well academically, and developing good reading skills, can be a great boost psychologically.

34

The Adolescent With Rheumatoid Arthritis

Ah, the joys of adolescence! Adolescence can be one of the most difficult periods in one's life. Adolescents are swingers, not because they have such active social lives (although they may), but because their behavior and moods may swing so extremely, from the childish dependence of years gone by to the mature independence of adult years approaching. Adolescents are frequently insecure and unstable. The adolescent years tend to be sensitive ones. Resentment and rebellion may arise when needs or desires are thwarted. Closeness is also possible on those occasions when adult understanding is shown. The adolescent usually works hard to become more independent, and asserts his or her independence in front of parents. Adolescents want to be on their own. They want to be able to stand up for themselves. At the same time, they don't want to be too different. JRA and its treatment can, in many cases, make them feel very different. This can create problems.

For young children, the restrictions of both JRA and its treatment may be unpleasant but tolerable. However, for adolescents living in their "glory days," they may be much more upsetting. Having to experience ongoing pain, seeing activities restricted, and feeling lethargic and unattractive, may be very depressing.

REBEL TIME

Finding out that an adolescent has JRA can cause major problems. The natural tendency of any parent is to become over-protective when a child is sick. Adolescents almost always object to interference from parents. Why? Because the adolescent wants to become more independent. The fact that parents frequently have difficulty dealing with any serious medical condition in their adolescent will, in all likelihood, increase adolescent rebellion. Rebellion is a normal part of adolescence, regardless of whether or not JRA is involved. Parents should try not to be overprotective, but as tolerant and understanding as possible. In cases where the adolescent does something wrong, supportive discussions are more appropriate than put-downs and reproaches.

Rebellion may occasionally lead to more serious physical problems for the adolescent. Why? Because a rebellious teenager may be less diligent with proper dietary maintenance. On occasion, the adolescent may deliberately try to make himself or herself worse, perhaps by not taking the proper medication or by doing too much (or too little). The adolescent knows that these behaviors can be harmful. So what? Hopefully, he or she will learn (without dangerous consequences) that there are better ways to get through adolescence!

PROBLEMS WITH FRIENDS

JRA may result in reductions in friendships. This can be a problem for anyone, but especially for the adolescent. Making friends is probably one of the most important activities during the adolescent years. Restrictions because of JRA reduce available activities. The adolescent may have a hard time deciding whether to tell friends, and if so, which ones? There may be concern that this information will hurt friendships, new or old. Parents need to be aware of this, so they can try to help. In rare cases, the adolescent might even want teachers to provide short classroom lessons about JRA, what it is and what it can do (after learning themselves, of course!) Hopefully, this will bring about more support and understanding.

EMBARRASSING!

Many adolescents are embarrassed about their condition. To an adolescent, any illness can be a stigma. Teenagers have to be "o.k." or it may cost them friends (so they believe). What about the stigma of having JRA? And what if JRA causes growth problems? It's hard to convince an unhappy adolescent with JRA that "good things come in small packages." Adolescents are at that stage in their lives when social relationships are the most important. They may be less able to get involved in physical activities or go to the gym. They may be more reluctant to develop social relationships because of concerns about "feeling different." All this may create a lot of discomfort in their young minds.

It should, therefore, be up to the adolescent to decide who he or she wants to tell. Teachers should probably know about the illness, since the adolescent may have certain needs or concerns that require more delicate attention. Why might the adolescent choose not to share this information with all friends? He or she might sense that, in some cases, friends would be afraid, upset, or even hostile. Some friends might ignore the adolescent, not wanting to be near someone with a chronic medical problem like JRA for fear they can "catch" it. So let your adolescent make the decision.

If the adolescent seems to be having too much difficulty coping with JRA, professional counseling may be helpful. Sometimes, an objective and supportive person can quickly get a troubled adolescent to learn how to adjust to an otherwise emotionally-painful disease.

WHO HANDLES IT BETTER?

Many adolescents with JRA cope better than their parents do! Parents may feel guilty. They may feel that *they* could have done something to prevent it. Parents frequently feel that it is their responsibility to protect their child from harm, disease, or injury. Remember: Adolescents who are involved in effective treatment can usually maintain fairly normal, active lives, despite JRA.

Occasionally, an adolescent may act differently with friends (and in school) than with parents or other family members. Could it be that the adolescent enjoys the protection and concern of parents? Maybe the adolescent puts on a different "face" with family than with friends. Isn't that frequently the case, even if JRA isn't involved? Adolescents may be more willing to confide in their parents than in friends. They don't want friends to think they complain all the time.

Some parents try to protect their adolescents by not telling them everything about their conditions. This is usually not the best approach. Adolescents should know the truth, so they can take responsibility for their own management. Adjusting to JRA may take a while. By restricting information, it may take even longer. Anger and bitterness between adolescents and their parents may seriously hurt the relationship.

QUESTIONING THE FUTURE

As the adolescent gets older, certain troublesome questions may come to mind. The adolescent may wonder, ''Will I be able to marry? . . . Will I be able to have children? . . . Will I be able to perform my job well enough to keep it? . . . Will I be able to make and keep friends? . . . Will I be able to finish my education? . . . Will I be able to function as a normal member of society? . . .'' These questions bother almost all adolescents. Having JRA just makes them more worrisome. The answers? As long as the new condition is taken into consideration, and lifestyle is adjusted where necessary, the adolescent with JRA should be in the same position to answer these questions as any other healthy teenager.

On To The Future

Well, you've just about finished this book. We've covered a lot of information about rheumatoid arthritis. However, it's nice to know that research continues to investigate ways of improving the effectiveness of treatment.

Tremendous progress has been made in treatment for RA. Earlier diagnosis has led to earlier, more effective treatment, resulting in a better prognosis. Ongoing research continues to test new drugs and techniques for treating the illness, as well as further improving the quality of life for the person with RA.

Perhaps by the time you read this, some drug or treatment may have proven itself to be more successful than ones currently available. For example, recent research has suggested that the use of fish oil may help control inflammation, and may decrease joint tenderness. It remains to be seen whether this, or other substances, will improve your life with RA. But at least people are working on the problem.

It will take time to determine how effective these procedures—and others—will be in the treatment of RA. In addition, it is hoped that scientists may soon discover other types of treatments that may entirely eliminate rheumatoid arthritis as a medical problem. Until then, hopefully you've learned a lot about how to cope with your RA. Although it would be impossible to include every possible problem that might be caused by RA, I hope that what you've read will help you to develop your own strategies for coping.

Because things change, and something that troubles you one day may not trouble you the next (and vice versa), use this book as a resource. Whenever you have questions about how to cope with a certain aspect of rheumatoid arthritis, consult these pages. If you have any comments—information you feel is important—or additional questions, feel free to write to me in care of the publisher. I'd be happy to hear from you. But for now, look brightly ahead, act proudly, and enjoy life as best you can. I wish all of my readers the very best of health and happiness!

Appendix

For further reading:

Lazarus, A. *In the Mind's Eye*. New York: Rawson Associates, 1977.

Linchitz, R. *Life Without Pain*. Reading, MA: Addison-Wesley Publishing Co., Inc., 1988.

For further information, contact:

Arthritis Foundation (National Office)
1314 Spring Street, N. W.
Atlanta, GA 30309

(404) 872-7100

National Chronic Pain Outreach
4922 Hampden Lane
Bethesda, MD 20814

(301) 652-4948

Index

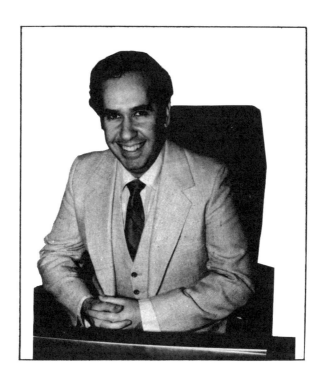

About the Author

Robert H. Phillips, Ph.D., is a practicing psychologist on Long Island, New York. He is the founder and director of the Center for Coping with Chronic Conditions, a multi-service organization helping individuals with chronic illness, and their families. He is involved with a number of local and national medical organizations. In addition, he is the psychologist for and director of the "Cope" program for the Long Island chapter of the Lupus Foundation of America, and is the associate director of the International Coma Recovery Institute.

The author of numerous articles on a variety of subjects in psychology, Dr. Phillips has lectured at conventions, universities, and professional meetings throughout the country, and has appeared on local and national radio and television programs.